Approaches to
the care of
adolescents

## DATE DUE

| | | | |
|---|---|---|---|
| NOV 2 2 '76 | | | |
| NOV 12 '76 | | | |
| FEB 20 '79 | | | |
| FEB 7 '79 | | | |
| JAN 12 1981 | | | |
| DEC 10 | | | |
| MAY 10 1981 | | | |
| MAY 17 1982 | | | |
| APR 2 2 1982 | | | |
| JAN 9 mar | | | |
| FEB 6 '84 | | | |
| FEB 3 1984 | | | |
| MAR 1 6 '87 | | | |
| FEB 23 '87 | | | |
| MAY 2 1996 | | | |
| 1/08/06 | | | |
| | | | |
| GAYLORD | | | |

D1260073

# APPROACHES TO

# THE CARE OF

# ADOLESCENTS

# APPROACHES TO THE CARE OF ADOLESCENTS

### EDITED BY

## AUDREY J. KALAFATICH, R.N., M.S.

*Associate Professor, Pediatric Nursing, University of Illinois, College of Nursing, Chicago, Illinois; Former Associate Professor And Program Director, Child Health Services, The Ohio State University School of Nursing, Columbus, Ohio*

### FOREWORD BY

## THOMAS E. SHAFFER, M.D.

APPLETON-CENTURY-CROFTS/New York
A Publishing Division of Prentice-Hall, Inc.

Library of Congress Cataloging in Publication Data
   Main entry under title:

   Approaches to the care of adolescents.

      Includes bibliographies and index.
      1.  Youth—Diseases.  2.  Youth—Health and hygiene.
   I.  Kalafatich, Audrey J., ed. [DNLM: 1.  Adolescence
   —Congresses.  2.  Comprehensive health care—
   Congresses.   WS460  A652  1971]
   RJ550.A66              616              74-19444
   ISBN  0-8385-0289-X

Copyright© 1975 by APPLETON-CENTURY-CROFTS
A Publishing Division of Prentice-Hall, Inc.

*All rights reserved. This book, or parts
thereof, may not be used or reproduced in
any manner without written permission. For
information address Appleton-Century-
Crofts, 292 Madison Avenue, New York,
N.Y. 10017*

75 76 77 78 79 / 10 9 8 7 6 5 4 3 2 1

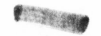

PRINTED IN THE UNITED STATES OF AMERICA

*Cover design by:  Johanna Cooper*

# Contributors

**SHIRLEY SMITH ASHBURN, R.N., M.S.**
*Instructor and Coordinator of Nursing Growth and Development Series, The Ohio State University School of Nursing, Columbus, Ohio*

**PATRICIA A. BRANDT, R.N., M.S.**
*Pediatric Nurse Specialist, The University of Utah College of Nursing, Salt Lake City, Utah; Maternal & Child Health Project, Shiprock Service Unit, Indian Health Service, Shiprock, New Mexico; Former Instructor in Pediatric Nursing, The Ohio State University School of Nursing (where she was involved with the terminally ill adolescent), Columbus, Ohio*

**NANCY M. BRUCE, A.C.S.W.**
*Social Worker, Adolescent Services, Columbus Children's Hospital, Columbus, Ohio*

**ALICE E. DAWSON, A.C.S.W.**
*Social Worker, Adolescent Services, Columbus Children's Hospital, Columbus, Ohio*

**FRANCIS W. EBERLY, M.D.**
*Associate Physician, University Health Service, The Ohio State University; Former Medical Director, The Teenage Clinic, Columbus Children's Hospital, Columbus, Ohio*

**JANET FENDER, R.N., B.S.**
*Public Health Nurse, Columbus, Ohio; (Senior nursing student at The Ohio State University School of Nursing at time of the study)*

**KAY FORSYTHE FENTON, R.N., B.S.**
*Head Nurse, Adolescent Psychiatric Unit, Upham Hall, Ohio State University Hospitals*

v

**ROBERT W. HERSHBERGER, R.N., M.S.**
*Director of Nursing, Bethesda Hospital, Zanesville, Ohio*

**AUDREY J. KALAFATICH, R.N., M.S.**
*Associate Professor, Pediatric Nursing, University of Illinois, College of Nursing, Chicago, Illinois; Former Associate Professor and Program Director, Child Health Care Services, The Ohio State University School of Nursing, Columbus, Ohio*

**ELAINE SCHROEDER, R.N., M.S.**
*Assistant Professor, Maternal-Child Nursing; Instructor, Lamaze Method of Childbirth Education, Capital University, Columbus, Ohio*

**THOMAS E. SHAFFER, M.D.**
*Associate Physician, University Health Services, The Ohio State University; Former Medical Director, The Teenage Clinic, Columbus Children's Hospital, Columbus, Ohio*

**JOHN N. STEPHENSON, M.D.**
*Director, The Teenage Clinic; Assistant Professor, Pediatrics; Assistant Professor, University Health Services, The University of Wisconsin, Madison, Wisconsin*

# Preface

This book on approaches to the care of adolescents was developed following a continuing education Workshop for nurses held at The Ohio State University in the fall, 1971. The purposes of the Workshop were to help the participants gain an in-depth understanding of who the adolescent is and some of the problems he faces as he grows to adulthood. In addition, the participants were helped to learn the therapeutic use of self in dealing with the adolescent who has entered some aspect of the health care system.

The enrollment for this Workshop far exceeded our expectations. Participation was excellent, and following the Workshop we had many requests for the papers presented and for any additional information related to the care of adolescents.

The faculty and guests who helped to present the Workshop discussed these requests among themselves and agreed that what was needed was a book written about the approaches to care for the adolescent. Although much has been written about theory of adolescent development and about causal and naturalistic observations of adolescents, none of the program participants were familiar with literature that handled the problems of adolescents in the same or a similar way in which they were handled in the Workshop, i.e., defining the problems and offering possible approaches.

All of the contributors to this book were faculty or students at The Ohio State University or affiliated in some way with the University or with Columbus Children's Hospital, at the time of the Workshop. The Hospital has a large, nationally known Teenage Clinic and several of the contributors work on a daily basis in direct contact with teenagers and their problems. Because of the excellent expertise of these people in this one geographic area, it was unnecessary to seek outside contributors.

This book was primarily written for the undergraduate nursing student, but should be useful to a much wider audience.

Graduate nursing students will find in the book a good overview of the adolescent and his problems and may use it as a starting point for a more detailed study of this age group. Because the book points out problems and possible approaches, the graduate nursing student should find ideas for clinical research.

In addition, public health nurses, school nurses, and staff nurses who must deal with adolescents in their every-day practice will find the book a useful reference.

Finally, although the book was written to fill the gap in the literature of adolescents and to be especially helpful to nurses, any member of any discipline who works with the adolescent will find much useful information. The nature of the problems of the adolescents makes the delivery of health care to this age group less clearly delineated in terms of who provides the care. Thus, medical students, social work students, student teachers, and counselors may find themselves involved with almost any of the kinds of problems dealt with in this book.

I would like to express my personal gratitude to the contributors. Although each one was actively involved in patient care in one way or another and each had his own personal commitments, they took the time to share their knowledge of adolescents and their experiences and then to write the chapters of this book. The contributors and I are also grateful to the adolescent patients with whom we have worked and from whom we have learned much.

Personal thanks are extended to Dr. Edna Menke, friend and colleague, for her support and assistance in the Project. I am also grateful to Rae Langford, one of my graduate students, for reading the manuscript and offering valuable comments. No project would ever reach completion without the expertise of a good secretary. I would especially like to recognize the contribution of Mrs. Diana Martin, who in addition to the many duties she performs as secretary, also typed the manuscript.

Audrey J. Kalafatich

# Contents

# Foreword

Although parents, poets, educators, social agencies, and court authorities have long been concerned about the problems of adolescents, these young people are just beginning to receive a full measure of the consideration and understanding they should have.

The interest others have had in adolescents was prophetic of the involvement with teenagers that health professionals have expressed in recent years. A generation ago adolescents were ordinarily regarded as being a group with few health problems. Serious physical illness is rare at this stage of life as is mortality from physical causes. Adolescents have usually been regarded as an "in-between" group, no longer really children and not quite adults, basically healthy, with few demands for scientifically administered health care. The surprising lack of interest in the medical care of adolescents was probably due to these facts, which indeed are deceptive. There has been an almost universal failure to recognize that minor health problems become major ones for adolescents when basic needs for independence, peer group recognition, and respect for their own identity are threatened by illness or disability. Apparently insignificant health problems will usually be viewed in an entirely different way by adolescents compared to children or adults.

In the light of our present perceptions about teenagers, present-day interest in the health care of adolescents is not surprising. Here is a large segment of the population, almost one-fifth of the total in our country, which appears to have good health, as estimated by ordinary measures. However, these supposedly healthy individuals often are the cause of concern in families and communities because of health-related problems—bizarre behavior, misuse of drugs, expression of sexuality, disinterest in school and apparent lack of motivation, foresight, and adjustability. As is often the case when there are deviations from what is considered to be "normal," physicians and other professionals in health care may well be the first to be consulted about personal problems of a general nature. The health care of adolescents thus becomes more than medical practice, and must include interest and familiarity in education, recreation, sports, and the social and psychologic aspects of adolescents' development as well as knowledge about typical health problems.

Those with an interest in adolescence come to recognize that this word signifies more than pubertal growth and maturation, with the accompanying problems of acne, obesity, dysmenorrhea, athletic injuries, and seizures. All of these do occur, but there must also be consideration for the adolescent's own feelings about growing, maturing, being "different," experiencing sexuality, and frequent concerns about what all of this has to do with eventually being an adult. So, a surge of interest in the health care of adolescents has occurred, influenced by realizations that those who become involved must always be alert to the psychologic and social significance as well as the physiologic and medical aspects of the problems that parents, educators, social agencies, and the adolescents themselves bring to the health specialists.

Thirty years ago medical textbooks and periodicals had very few references to adolescents. Most of those which could be found dealt with behavioral and educational topics. The big health issues defined as medical, social, or psychologic require consideration of every aspect of adolescent growth and development. This is the challenge. The goal is being met by interdisciplinary conferences, postgraduate courses, seminars, and the mushrooming growth of comprehensive health centers for adolescents. Not enough of the products from these endeavors reach others who could use them. Those who can do the most for adolescents are at the operational level where services are being given. For this reason it is a happy occasion when Miss Kalafatich and her collaborators have made available to a wide audience the facts and philosophy which were presented at a conference on the health care of adolescents.

Thomas E. Shaffer, M.D.

# APPROACHES TO

# THE CARE OF

# ADOLESCENTS

# 1

# Adolescence –
# A Separate Stage of Life

AUDREY J. KALAFATICH

Opinions and thoughts about what a teenager is vary according to the perceiver's interest, background, and experience. Each reader, I'm sure, has his or her own thoughts on the subject. For purposes of clarification, we shall define a teenager as an individual in that stage of development between childhood and adulthood—no longer considered a child, he is not yet an adult. He is experiencing biologic, physiologic, and psychologic changes. Moreover, a particular level of social behavior is required of him, one more complex than that of childhood but not yet that allowed the adult.[1]

Adolescence is indeed a stage separate and unique along life's continuum. In working with teenagers, it is necessary to understand where the youngster has been on this continuum and where he is going in order to understand him now. One aspect of this continuum is psychologic development.

Erikson[2](p 1) divides the psychologic development of an individual through the life cycle into eight stages (Table 1). Adolescence is the fifth of these, so that the adolescent already has dealt with four of them.

**Table 1**

**ERIKSON'S STAGES OF DEVELOPMENT**

1. Trust vs. mistrust
2. Autonomy vs. shame and doubt
3. Initiative vs. guilt
4. Industry vs. inferiority
5. Identity vs. role confusion
6. Intimacy and solidarity vs. isolation
7. Generativity vs. self-absorption
8. Integrity vs. despair

According to Erikson, the first stage of psychosocial development centers around the belief "I am what I am given," the second, "I am what I will." Characteristically, the third stage features "I am what I imagine I will be" and the fourth, "I am what I learn."[2](p 82) This, then, is what the individual brings with him to adolescence, wherein he forms his crucial sense of identity. Adolescence is therefore critical for Erikson's three stages of adulthood. From his schema it follows that the individual must establish a reasonable sense of identity before he can become intimate (the sixth stage) with any other person, especially a member of the opposite sex.[2](p 95) In the seventh stage, generativity, the individual deals with guidance of the next generation so that, again, his own sense of identity is essential or prerequisite. The eighth stage, integrity, deals with the acceptance of one's own life style, but this is crystallized during the identity stage of adolescence.

Thus, although true that the teenager is no longer a child, he *does* bring all-important childhood experiences to this stage. And though not yet an adult, many youngsters at this stage think about what it means to be an adult. A common admonition directed by adults toward teenagers is to "Act your age!" Most of the time, the teenager is doing just that! And clearly the teenager's "age" is a period that is decisive for his later development.

Adolescence, then, is a psychologic, social, and maturational process characterized by rapid growth, both physical and psychologic.[1] Note that I use the word "process." "Process" implies change, something that is ongoing. Those of us who deal with adolescents can readily vouch for this as we know that people at this age are certainly changing and changeable. We shall now look at these characteristics of teenagers in more detail. They are divided into biologic, psychologic, and social aspects, and are interrelated. For discussion purposes, however, we shall examine each separately.

Biologically, at puberty and during early adolescence the youngster's body increases in height and weight. He is growing and must therefore learn to adapt to his changing and subsequently larger body. Because skeletal maturation exceeds muscle ability, the discrepancy between skeletal growth and muscle development produces awkwardness in most teenagers even though manual dexterity is good. And since physical maturity is reached before psychologic maturity, the individual *looks* like an adult long before he can be expected to act like one. Other physical changes are the development of primary and secondary sex characteristics.

In girls, the development of the breasts is one of the earliest manifestations of beginning sexual maturation during normal puberty. These breast changes are followed by the appearance of pubic hair, menstruation, and axillary hair, in that order. That adolescent girls are conscious and also self-conscious of these changes is demonstrated in the following example.

Three of us, Denise, a fourteen-year-old, the medical intern who was doing an admission physical examination on her, and myself, were in an examining room on a hospital ward. Denise was wearing her pajama top backwards with the buttons down the back during the examination. When the examination was completed, the intern told her that she could dress and return to her room. When I offered to help her turn the pajama top around, she refused my help and proceeded to turn it around in a way that did not expose her breasts. She seemed embarrassed at the prospect of exposing them and obviously took pains to avoid this.

In addition to the above-mentioned physical changes in body shape in girls, also their hips widen, giving the girl a more feminine hourglass shape.

In boys the onset of puberty is signified by an increase in the size of the testes and penis and an expansion of the shoulders and chest. In some of my work with very young teenage boys, I found that they sometimes measure their penises and compare its size and consider the size to be a mark of "manliness." I have also had boys ask me to measure their urine outputs; and they kept a record of these for 24-hour periods. I never discussed their requests with them, but I felt these were in some way a competitive venture and, again, a test of "manliness."

Other biologic changes in adolescence are alterations in the body's physiology. Most significant of these and one sometimes used to determine onset of adolescence is sexual maturation—that is, the ability to reproduce. This is defined by menstruation in girls although it does not follow that girls are capable of reproduction at the onset of menstruation. In boys sexual maturation is more difficult to determine but is based on the presence of fertile spermatozoa. Although the manifestation appears to be abrupt in both sexes, the onset actually is gradual. Female hormones from the anterior pituitary gland stimulate the production of hormones in the ovaries and thus stimulate menarche. A similar type of endocrine activity in boys stimulates growth of the testes and prostatic activity, and thus the production of sperm. Another physiologic alteration at puberty and during adolescence is increased perspiration and increased secretion from the sebaceous glands. The latter may result in acne.

Several authors state that the psychologic tension present during the adolescent period is brought about by the above physiologic changes.[3-5] No studies could be found in the literature which documented this belief. The changing body does however bring about one of the major tasks of adolescence, which is the acceptance of one's own changing body.[6-9] The fact of "having a body that changes, of being a body in the process of change, cannot help drawing the attention of the individual toward his changing body . . . "[9]

Two widely accepted theories concerning tasks related to adolescence are those of Erikson and Havighurst. As mentioned previously, Erikson divides the psychosexual development of an individual through the life cycle into eight stages, where each stage represents a crisis which can be dealt with in one of two ways (Table 1, p. 2). The tasks are worked on during each stage and some resolution of them is achieved by the end of each.

According to Erikson, the adolescent faces the task of establishing ego identity versus the possibility of role confusion. Erikson defines this sense of ego identity as "the accrued confidence that one's ability to maintain inner sameness and continuity (one's ego in the psychologic sense) is matched by the sameness and continuity of one's meaning for others." Failure to achieve this sense of identity results in role confusion.[2 (p 53)]

According to Havighurst[7(pp 33-62)] the developmental tasks for the adolescent arise from individual needs and societal demands. Individual needs include such things as accepting one's own body and learning to use it effectively. Societal demands call for the adolescent to achieve socially responsible behavior, which includes the attaining of independence from parents and the achieving of a masculine or feminine social role. Havighurst's developmental tasks of adolescence are as follows:

1. achieving emotional independence of parents and other adults
2. achieving assurance of economic independence
3. selecting and preparing for an occupation
4. preparing for marriage and family life
5. developing intellectual skills and concepts necessary for civic competence
6. desiring and achieving socially responsible behavior
7. acquiring a set of values and an ethical system as a guide to behavior
8. achieving new and more mature relations with age mates of both sexes
9. achieving a masculine or feminine social role
10. accepting one's physique and using one's body effectively[12](pp 33–62)

That the search for identity is a major task of adolescence is well supported in the literature. Deutsch says that the question: "Am I a man or a woman?" is of major concern to the adolescent girl.[10] Blos concurs with the idea that girls (more often than boys) are much more consciously occupied by the idea: Am I a boy or a girl? Blos further contends that "often girls maintain the belief that they can decide either way . . . "[11]

Jeanette, a thirteen-year-old with scoliosis, demonstrated very little interest in her feminine identity. On admission to the hospital, she did not look like the "typical" female teenager. For example, she did have long hair but did not seem particularly interested in its grooming. In conversation she expressed negative feelings about her feminine identity and even seemed skeptical about it. After she had had her hair cut very short in preparation for the application of a body cast, she exclaimed: "I look like a boy!" She seemed to imply that the haircut, which made her look like a boy, might have, in fact, transformed her into one.

English and Pearson also imply a search for the individual's identity in stating that "an important conflict that the individual has to work out during adolescence is between his desire to be regarded as an adult and his wish to remain a child."[12]

Although the search for an identity and the acceptance of one's changing body is a major task of adolescence, there is general agreement that the most important developmental task is giving up childhood ties and achieving a degree of independence. Deutsch notes that during prepuberty and puberty, the life cycle periods just preceding adolescence, the young girl has a strong need to free herself from her mother and from dependence on her.[10] Deutsch further contends that the young girl wants to achieve adulthood without her mother's help. However, emotional ties to the mother persist and emotions are often transferred to a mother substitute; that is, to another adult, such as a teacher or nurse. Because she is trying to free herself from her mother, the young girl may not want to have anything to do with her. By completely renouncing mother, the young girl may feel that she can better sever the tie.

Separation, and thus a degree of independence, would seem to be easier for boys since the same strong emotional tie that occurs between girls and their mothers does not seem to occur with boys. Childrearing practices in this country are such that girls are reared in such a way as to be closely tied to mother, whereas boys are not.

Josselyn agrees that the adolescent must sever childhood ties and that, when faced with unfamiliar elements within the environment, must turn to others for support.[13] The other person that the adolescent turns to usually is some adult other than a parent. However, the adolescent "resents this dependency because it threatens his confidence in himself as a potential adult."[13(p 51)] He resents his inability to be totally independent and vents his anger on those who are aware of his inadequacies—parents and other adults. This major task of adolescence, the struggle for independence, involves the reorganization of emotional ties which is begun by an almost total rejection of any attachment to parents and other adults.[1(p 66)] The adolescent learns to revise his patterns of functioning, especially in the areas of emotional attachment and in his ways of thinking. In other words, he learns to act and think for himself.

One of the methods used by the adolescent to handle the psychologic stress incurred by this struggle for independence is strenuous physical activity in work or play.[10(p 5),14] Physical activity seems to be a way of purging the body of pent-up emotions and feelings that the adolescent is reluctant to discharge in any other way. Physical activity also gives the adolescent the impression that he is in control. According to Ausubel:[14]

> Motor ability of an individual during adolescence . . . constitutes an important component of his feeling of competence in coping with the environment. It enables him to be competent and capable of meeting his own needs . . . physical activity continues to provide an important source of personal satisfaction, pleasure, relaxation, and leisure time activity. (p 20)

Deutsch states that in addition to the positive aspects of the use of activity, adolescent girls also use activity in the form of flight in their attempts to free themselves from the strong emotional ties of childhood.[10] Deutsch says that "one of the less commendable methods of breaking the tie with the parental home, and one that is frequently used in puberty, is actual flight." She concludes that flight ultimately may lead to more tension as the individual adolescent must, sooner or later, either return to the home or remain cut off from those close to her. The use of flight is also seen in boys in such activities as athletics, driving cars, and so forth.

Another important psychosocial characteristic of the

adolescent is his dependency upon his peer group. [1][3(p 39)] The peer group is composed of individuals at approximately the same level of emotional development and serves as a support as well as a testing ground for the individual adolescent.[1(p 68)] The peer group helps its members to cope with changing bodies by offering a comparison group and, in the same way, helps them to handle their strivings for independence. Each member of the group is able to compare his own relationships with parents and other adults with the way other members of the group handle similar relationships.

In summary, adolescence is indeed a "separate stage of life." It is a biologic, physiologic, and psychologic process during which changes are expected in social behavior. Changes in the body's physical structure and in its physiologic functions normally occur at this time. Body structure is altered by increases in height and weight, and by growth and development of muscles. The adolescent gets bigger and develops greater coordination. Body structure is also altered by the appearance of secondary sex characteristics. While the body changes externally, internal changes also are taking place. Growth of the primary sex characteristics occurs, namely, the organs of reproduction. These physical and physiologic changes, including changes in hormone production, result in changes in body functioning.

The major psychosocial tasks of adolescence include the achieving of a sense of identity and the achieving of a degree of independence in preparation for assuming an adult role in society. The adolescent must answer for himself the question "Who am I?" In so doing, he must redefine his roles for himself, especially his roles with his parents and family.

Lastly, the importance of the "adult friend" and the significance of the peer group were discussed. The peer group is especially important to the individual in helping him to master the tasks of adolescence.

REFERENCES

1. Committee on Adolescence, Group for the Advancement of Psychiatry: Normal Adolescence: Its Dynamics and Impact. New York, Scribner's, 1968
2. Erikson EH: Identity and the life cycle. Psychol Issues, Monogr 1, 1:1, 1959
3. Rabinovitch R: Psychology of adolescence. Pediatr Clin North Am Vol 8, Feb 1960, pp 65—83
4. Heald FP: Medical problems of the adolescent. Panel report, Current Medical Digest 33:2, Feb 1966, pp 189—249
5. Gallagher JR, Harris HI: Emotional Problems of Adolescence. New York, Oxford U Press, 1958
6. Hurlock EB: Adolescent Development, 3rd ed. New York, McGraw-Hill, 1969, p 56
7. Havighurst RJ: Development Tasks and Education, 2nd ed. New York, McKay, 1952
8. Horrocks JE: The Psychology of Adolescence, 3rd ed. Boston, Houghton, 1969, p 342
9. Oesterrieth PA: Adolescence: some psychosocial aspects. In Caplan G, Lebovici S (eds): Adolescence: Psychosocial Perspectives. New York, Basic Books, 1969, pp 11—21
10. Deutsch H: The Psychology of Women, Vol 1: Girlhood. New York, Grune & Stratton, 1944, p 86
11. Blos P: On Adolescence. New York, Free Press of Glencoe, 1962, p 83
12. English S, Pearson GHJ: Emotional Problems of Living. New York, Norton, 1955, p 323
13. Josselyn I: The Adolescent and His World. New York, Family Service Association of America, 1952, pp 47—51
14. Ausubel DP: Theory and Problems of Adolescent Development. New York, Grune & Stratton, 1954


BIBLIOGRAPHY

Caplan G, Lebovici S (eds): Adolescence: Psychosocial Perspectives. New York, Basic Books, 1969
Committee on Adolescence, Group for the Advancement of Psychiatry: Normal Adolescence: Its Dynamics and Impact. New York, Scribner's, 1968
Deutsch H: Selected Problems of Adolescence. The Monograph Series of the Psychoanalytic Study of the Child, No 3. New York, International Universities Press, 1967

Eisenberg L: A developmental approach to adolescence. Children 12:4, July—August, 1965, pp 131—135

Erikson EH: Identity and the life cycle. Psychol Issues, Monogr 1, 50:1, 1959, p 53

Havighurst RJ: Developmental Tasks and Education, 2nd ed. New York, McKay, 1952

Horrocks JE: The Psychology of Adolescence, 3rd ed. Boston, Houghton, 1969

Hurlock EB: Adolescent Development, 3rd ed. New York, McGraw-Hill, 1969

Jersild AT: Psychology of Adolescence, 2nd ed. New York, Macmillan, 1963

Josselyn I: The Adolescent and His World. New York, Family Service Association of America, 1952

# 2

# The Health Care System – How Do Teenagers Use It?

SHIRLEY SMITH ASHBURN

The purpose of this chapter is to describe how teenagers use selected types of subsystems within the health care system in our society today. This information is based on a review of the literature in various disciplines as well as interviews with professionals. Included in this chapter are brief descriptions of selected subsystems and the majority of problems that teenagers bring to these. Other specific problems that are characteristic of many of the adolescent clients who use the health care system will be dealt with in more detail in forthcoming chapters. Effective approaches used in communicating with them and their families will be discussed.

## THE HEALTH CARE SYSTEM—WHAT KINDS OF SUBSYSTEMS EXIST FOR TEENAGERS TO USE?

Numerous health care subsystems exist that teenagers can use. They can, for example, often utilize the services offered to other age groups by private physicians, public health nurses, neighborhood clinics, outpatient clinics, school nurses, dentists, gynecologists, dermatologists, hospitals, and emergency rooms.

Just what brings teenagers to the health care system? While participating as a panel member during an Ohio State University continuing education workshop on adolescence, Dr. Thomas E. Shaffer reported on a study conducted in New York City to ascertain the chief complaints of adolescents who used the services of the hospital emergency room. According to Dr. Shaffer, those who came only once to the emergency room under study did so because of what was deemed a medical crisis (eg, the cramping pain associated with a genitourinary infection, or a broken leg during football practice). Those adolescents who returned more than once to the emergency room that was observed reported that they did so because of the positive interpersonal relations they experienced. It is this type of rapport that is essential in working with adolescents, especially within the subsystems that compose the health care system.

In addition to the well-known health care subsystems, there are those designed especially for teenage use. The following is a brief description of four selected subsystems that have programs for making the teenager feel accepted as a person.

The *private physician who specializes in adolescent medicine* is an excellent example. These pediatricians have elected to limit their clientele to adolescents (and often work closely with their families whenever the need arises). Teenagers are usually seen by these doctors on an appointment basis for a variety of reasons. These doctors may also be found in various types of clinics that are especially designed for teenagers.

Other health professionals who specialize in the care of adolescents also work in *teenage clinics*. These facilities are located both in hospital settings as outpatient clinics and also in various neighborhoods ("satellite clinics" of the hospital-based type.) Rigg and Fisher found thirty such adolescent outpatient facilities existing in the United States and Canada as of January 1958.[1 (p193)] The hospital-based clinics are either areas within a hospital specifically set aside for adolescents or are listed times on a hospital clinic's schedule specifically reserved for them. Although most of these clinics had only part-time physicians, nineteen of them had at least one full-time practitioner and sixteen had full-time resident physicians or fellows. Three of these clinics had full-time staff psychiatrists, and eighteen had at least one part-time psychiatrist. Some had public health nurses available in addition to other health workers, such as psychologists, social workers, and nutritionists, to work with adolescents.

Fortunately, more clinics for adolescents have opened since the Rigg and Fisher study. In 1970, fifty clinics designed especially for adolescents and staffed by people with the ability and desire to help this particular age group were operating in the United States.[2 (p 68)] Mount Sinai Hospital in New York City has an adolescent clinic which does much work with schools and social agencies in the area, such as the Youth Employment Service and the East Harlem Health Council.[2 (p 68)] Columbus Children's Hospital in Columbus, Ohio, has several "satellite clinics" that are branches of the Department of Health, Education and Welfare. Costs of care are based on the ability of the adolescent or his family to pay.

There is another type of community adolescent clinic which exists that is not directly associated with a hospital.

These *free clinics* are also staffed by doctors, nurses, social workers, and other allied health professionals. One of the secrets to their success in establishing the trust of their patients seems to be the fact that many are staffed with young volunteers who understand the problems of the teenagers in that community. An example of such a clinic is the Open Door Clinic in Columbus, Ohio, funded by the Columbus Area Community Mental Health Association, Franklin County 648 Board, and by private donations. Located as it is near the Ohio State University, many teenagers seek counsel and treatment there about some of their problems. Appointments are not necessary and arrangements are made for "on-call" counselling services during the hours that the clinic is formally closed. Staff from Open Door Clinic visit local public schools to discuss drugs, venereal disease, and problem pregnancy, factually and openly.

In addition to the two types of clinics, an increasing number of hospitals have established as separate medical care facilities for adolescents the *teenage unit.* The reason for having a teenage unit is not because teenagers have diseases that are unique; rather, because their psychosocial needs are different from those of other phases of the life cycle.

Advantages of these units include the fact that the staff, dealing solely with adolescents, can be prepared more easily to understand the differing manifestations of illness which appear during adolescence. In addition, the staff is also able to assist the individual teenager through periods of stress that teenagers generally may perceive as physically traumatizing.[3(p 37)] Teenagers also gain the benefit of being with others of their peer group. And they often are asked to aid in making and in enforcing rules for the unit. So important is this concept of a special unit for adolescents that the Committee on Hospital Practice Bed-Care of the Society of Adolescent Medicine has issued a comprehensive report with recommendations for physical organization of the unit, personnel, unit routine, and funding. Such recommendations include a unit with a recreation area (to accommodate group activities), "snack" bar (to provide the large amount of extra nutrition needed in adolescence for healing and growing, as well as serve as a focal point for socializing), and plenty of available telephones (to keep up the teenage lines of communication!).[4](p 18)

## COMMON HEALTH CONCERNS OF THE ADOLESCENT— WHO DO THEY SEE ABOUT THEM?

More and more teenagers are seeking assistance from the health care system, whether this be from a private doctor, clinic, school nurse, visiting public health nurse, or hospital. Dr. Thomas E. Shaffer, Professor of Pediatrics at The Ohio State University and noted authority on adolescent medicine, stated in his address to professionals at a 1971 workshop on adolescents that one-fifth of the U.S. population is between the ages of 10 and 19. He went on to hypothesize that perhaps the reason more teenagers are being assisted by health professionals today is that their generation is a more expressive one and, although they express their needs in different ways, they value help.

Having just returned from a meeting of the American Academy of Pediatrics, Dr. Shaffer reported that in comparison with most other age groups the mortality rate among teenagers is low. And their morbidity rate is also relatively low. Only the rate for accidental death and injury shows an increase in this segment of the population.[5](p 540) However, the emotional uncertainty attributed to this phase of the life cycle very much affects the adolescents who do have disorders and concerns. The following are a few of these disorders and concerns that pose real threats of physical and emotional disability to the adolescent. Significant signs and symptoms described in medical texts are included. Also mentioned are the most common health care subsystems and professionals who aid the adolescent in coping with the problem.

### Short-Term Problems of the Teenager

Skin disorders occur in both sexes so commonly in late childhood and during adolescence that they can almost be considered a normal aspect of sexual development.[6 (p 142)] The more apparent and disfiguring conditions, such as *acne* and *eczema*, cause the adolescent considerable embarrassment and discomfort and, as a result, often come to the attention of the school nurse. For those problems not attended to by school nurses, teenagers usually continue to treat these skin troubles by "home remedies" or patent preparations. Sometimes the peer group grapevine will endorse getting help at the neighborhood clinic. Unless the situation becomes unbearable to the individual, it is often the parent who guides the adolescent to seek the services of a private doctor.

Ear piercing is very popular among young girls because their friends are having it done and the practice is a part of their culture. Unfortunately, if the procedure is not safely performed by a professional or if the recipient does not adhere to principles of good hygiene, *ear piercing complications* may arise. Such complications include metal allergic dermatitis, crust formation, inflammation, bleeding, or cyst or belois formation. To protect against these complications, young girls who have diabetes, a history of belois formation, or skin disorders should have their ears pierced only by a physician, and after parental consent.[7 (p 702)]

Other teenager needs for professional help may be for *hearing, vision,* or *dental problems.* Sometimes these difficulties are detected by a school nurse.

Food faddism and poor eating habits of adolescents may result in *malnutrition* even in those whose families can financially afford an "adequate" diet. Private and clinic professionals state that adolescents tell them they eat this way because the diet promises to help them reduce, because it is popular or simple, or because it promises beauty or strength. Diet improvement usually ensues in a clinic where teenagers are offered the opportunity to discuss in small peer groups the necessity of a well-balanced diet. Also, private physicians and their nurses often give helpful literature concerning nutrition to the patient, in addition to discussing the teenager's diet with him individually.

Many teenagers frequently complain of *feeling tired*. Upon examination and the taking of a medical history, health professionals find that the causes of these fatigue sensations are extremely rapid physical growth, overactivity, lack of sleep, faulty nutrition, or an emotional problem. Any adolescent who exhibits persistent fatigue may be suffering from *anemia*. The teenager who has such complaints, especially if accompanied by fainting, pallor, poor appetite, or irritability, certainly should not be treated as a hypochondriac but as a patient with a physical problem.[6(p 94)]

*Obesity* is relatively common during the teenage years in both sexes. It is more frequent in the lower socioeconomic classes and often not brought to the attention of health professionals since many families consider it a normal part of "growing up."[5(p 78)] Health professionals in all settings are usually consulted about the problem either when the teenager can no longer cope with his threatening body image and/or a parent becomes concerned. (Approaches to obesity in teenage girls are presented in Chapter 5.)

*Gynecomastia* is another disorder especially ego-deflating to the male teenager. This hormonally induced enlargement of mammary tissue is embarrassing to the boys and health professionals constantly must reassure them that the condition is not serious and is transient.

*Irregular menstruation* and simple *menstrual disorders* deeply concern teenage girls. School nurses, clinic professionals, and private physicians often treat these difficulties and explain their meaning to the young patient.

Another hormonally induced phenomenon is an adolescent *goiter*, an enlargement of the thyroid gland due to the accelerated growth typical of early adolescence. Teenagers need to be helped to understand that the enlargement usually regresses spontaneously within a year or two.

Adolescents are normally very active. Often, when a *heart murmur* is heard during a routine physical examination, the physician must be careful not to become unnecessarily concerned and immediately suggest a restriction of activity. Since congenital heart disease is usually noticed before the teenage years, the majority of systolic murmurs heard in adolescents are functional. Of course these murmurs must be differentiated from more serious cardiac conditions, but care must be taken not to make the patient a "cardiac cripple."[6(p 107)]

Finally there is the condition of *faulty posture*, the cause of which is the common slow growth of muscles that young teenagers often experience. Health professionals need to stress that, as far as the physical needs of the adolescent are concerned, the only treatment for this condition is waiting for growth and, thus, strength to occur.

## Long-Term Conditions of the Teenager

Rapid body growth and development of the organs and functions of reproduction are the most significant physical changes that occur during adolescence.[6(p 64)] It is this onset of growth, however, that varies so markedly among individuals, and some experience temporary *growth failures*.

The school nurse is in an excellent position to detect such *growth failures* which may be the result of underweight. Hammer and Eddy state that 20 percent of teenagers are underweight.[6(p 64)] If nothing can be done to correct the condition, supporting facts are sometimes the best treatment that can be given to the boy who is slow to grow as tall as his peers, or the girl who "towers" over her feminine friends. The same principle must often be applied in working with the adolescent who is worried about not maturing sexually as fast as the rest of the peer group. In more serious cases, surgery and hormonal therapy must be used to treat these disorders.[8](p 1676)

*Scoliosis,* the S-shaped lateral curvature usually associated with rotation of the spine, is most frequent between the ages of 12 and 16, a period of rapid growth.[7](p 718) Functional scoliosis can be corrected by use of good postural practices. Only the more serious structural scoliosis requires physiotherapy and/or surgery.

*Chronic ulcerative colitis* often has its earliest onset during adolescence. Due to the seriousness of this disorder, more than one group of health care system professionals may be needed to treat the patient. The school nurse needs to work with the patient because prolonged absences from school are often caused by cyclic remissions and exacerbations; a doctor and nurse team familiar with the patient and his family is needed to treat these exacerbations; and a clinical psychologist or psychiatrist may be called in to aid the adolescent and his family in coping with the situation. Probably with no other disease is continuity of care more vital to the well-being of the patient. Ironically, the usually emotionally immature adolescent with ulcerative colitis responds best the fewer the number of persons with whom he must deal.[6](p 99)

Although the incidence of *tuberculosis* has decreased in the more advanced countries, it is still prevalent in underdeveloped, overcrowded areas. Adolescents seem more susceptible to tuberculosis than persons in other age groups.[7](p 716) Health professionals in emergency settings (eg, Red Cross immediate care) as well as those more permanent (eg, hospitals) must work to educate the patients on the treatment of tuberculosis as well as preventing its reinfection.

*Diabetes mellitus* during the teenage years can be a stressful disorder. Medication, diet, and activity adjustments must fluctuate with the rapid periods of growth that adolescents experience. Feeling comfortable enough to discuss his thoughts openly with an understanding doctor and nurse is of utmost importance for the patient. Should hospitalization be necessary, this need for understanding on behalf of all the staff is a must.

*Seizure disorders* are very common among children and adolescents. It has been postulated that the increased incidence of this disorder in adolescence may be related to some of the hormonal and physiologic changes that occur during this period of rapid growth.[6 (p 108)] Adjustments to this chronic illness are not easy. If healthy coping is to be established, the physician and nurse must work closely with the adolescent in anticipating problems that may arise in such areas as automobile driving, careers and vacations, and pregnancy.

*Unwed adolescent parenthood*, according to Marlow, occurs at every social, economic, and intellectual level, although most often the teenager who is seen by a public health worker has been socially and economically deprived.[7 (p 725)] (Approaches to pregnancy in teenagers are discussed in Chapter 3.)

*Alcoholism* can be likened to drug dependence. Teenagers can develop a physiologic addiction along with a psychologic compulsion for alcohol. *Drug dependence or abuse*, also prevalent among teenagers, is discussed in Chapter 7 at length.

Depending on their degree of *mental retardation*, adolescents who have this developmental disability will come in contact with various health care professionals. These range from the physician who can medically treat the cause of mental retardation to care furnished in an institution.

Hammer and Eddy state that most teenagers can learn to control an *asthma* condition through the use of drugs, the control of environmental irritants, and with desensitization. Public health nurses are able to carefully screen the asthma patient's home for factors which may be precipitating the attacks. Sometimes these include emotional factors, and health care professionals must therefore work closely with the adolescent and his family.[6][(p 96)]

Mildly *neurotic symptoms* are present in many adolescents. Most of these worries are caused by the challenges that adolescents face in our competitive society. A health professional who has established a good rapport with the adolescent and has gained his trust can usually treat this young individual successfully. When there is the possibility of deeper difficulties, however, a psychiatrist should be consulted.

Adolescents in great need of professional help are those who turn to deviant behavior (*juvenile delinquency*) as a way of coping with life. These individuals and often their families are ordered by court to seek aid at mental health clinics.

Some disturbed adolescents turn upon the world; others turn upon themselves. *Suicidal attempts* and *suicide* are not rare in adolescence (Chap. 9).

This concludes our discussion of the common disorders of adolescence. Many of them can be prevented. It goes without saying that preventive education and anticipatory guidance as goals for the understanding health professional can accomplish much with the typically conscientious teenager. It is this understanding—this "getting through to"—that is so important in working with teenagers who need health guidance.

## THE IMPORTANCE OF UNDERSTANDING THE TEENAGER— HOW IS THIS UNDERSTANDING USED BY HEALTH PROFESSIONALS?

Although it is true that certain medical conditions occur frequently during the adolescent years, adolescents are essentially a healthy group. Because of this fact, according to Dr. William A. Daniel, Jr., adolescents have been neglected medically. Dr. Daniel further states that the chief reason why general practitioners, pediatricians, and internists need to seek to learn more about adolescents is that these young people differ both physiologically and psychologically from children and adults.[9 (p 3)]

I believe this better understanding of adolescents should be the goal of all who come in contact with them—professionals and nonprofessionals alike. Parents have always expressed a desire to better understand their teenaged family members (and vice versa!). The successful teacher is the one who can communicate with the teenager because he is interested in understanding him. But to have gone through adolescence and experienced it does not by any means make one an expert on the subject.

It is often the professionals, however, that are called upon for guidance by the teenagers. Troubled teenagers may subconsciously seek the answers to their emotional problems by initially approaching a health professional with a presenting physical symptom. Complaints of "headache" or "stomach ache," for example, may have teenage worries and other problems of a more personal nature as their origin. These underlying problems are most often finally expressed to the health care professional who takes the time to establish a trusting relationship with the teenager.

Daubenmire et al[10] found in their study of hospitalized adolescents that those who did seek information from hospital personnel most frequently chose the nurse. It cannot be assumed that the nurse is capable of completely making illness and hospitalization a more positive experience for the adolescent. Rather, it is anticipated that, as a result of the nurse-patient relationship, the adolescent can find sufficient expression to unleash psychologic forces and move toward emotional growth. This principle applies to all health professionals who successfully interact with adolescents.

It is important to mention at this point that one must be cautious in assuming that, just because a patient is an adolescent, he has emotional problems. Conway quotes Kuhlen in stating that care must be taken not to create problems by looking for them, yet one must be sensitive to the possibility that they may exist.[11 (p 77)]

In a time of increasing depersonalization, though, how do you communicate with a teenager? In a "course-happening" involving adolescents and adults at the University of California, the following requirements were summarized as necessary for effective intergenerational dialogue:[12 (p 223)]

1. To be willing to listen and to hear
2. To guide, but not to goad, others
3. To be open-minded
4. To be innovative rather than imitative
5. To act rather than to react
6. To care enough to try

Carrying out such techniques as these have greatly aided the interpersonal relations between health professionals and teenagers. For example, Mrs. Kathy Dufrane, a nurse at one of the Columbus Children's Hospital satellite clinics, states that her policy concerning patients who break appointments is not a punishing one. Rather, she sends a message expressing concern, communicating an "I'm interested in you" attitude. In other words, she attempts to guide the patient back to the clinic, not "goad" him into coming back. When the individual does come back, she makes it a point to listen with an open mind to whatever he has to say. There are times when a teenager's values differ from her own, but as long as the young person does not medically harm himself, she does not try to impose any external values on him. Most teenagers are quite conscious of what others think of them for this feeds into their self-concept. Obviously, Mrs. Dufrane's approach could aid a teenager to feel that he is recognized and respected as an individual.

One of the common concerns of adolescents is the question, "Am I growing up the way I should?" Teenagers having this concern about their body image do not feel relieved when someone tells them "not to worry" or that "nothing is wrong." As Dr. Morgenthau at Mount Sinai says about a fifteen-year-old boy who worried about being "too short, . . . there isn't much you can tell a youngster like this except that his growth will probably come sooner or later. But just being able to talk about it to someone, to recognize that the problem exists, unburdens the teenager's mind."[2(p 70)]

In working with the adolescent patient, the teaching principle of beginning where the student is can be applied. This includes assessing the teenager's biopsychosocial needs since the adolescent's emotional age may not correlate with his chronologic age. Furthermore, if today's young person is a member of a minority group, such as Negro, Indian, or Mexican-American, or if his parents or grandparents come from Puerto Rico or Japan, adolescence and the developmental tasks required by our society can appear even more painful for them. One therefore must strive to treat the individual adolescent in terms of who he is—an *individual.*

Keeping all of this in mind, the health professional must also remember that fear often causes minor discomfort to become intensified into a painful situation.[13(p 127)] Therefore, explanations of his medical problem that the adolescent is capable of understanding are in order. These explanations do not have to be childlike; teenagers usually enjoy learning about themselves and want to know the medical terminology that is being used to describe their case. It is important, however, that the teaching health professional should in some way request feedback from the young listener to assure that the patient is not so anxious as to distort the necessary information he is receiving.

There are many times when it is not enough for the teenager to have someone who will listen or someone with whom he can talk; he feels the need to be doing something to help himself. Emotions can be constructively channeled by linking high level wellness goals with the teenager's interests and hobbies. For example, if a young adolescent girl with diabetes is an avid reader, she can be encouraged to read more about diabetes. If she is interested in sewing or art, she may make various containers for storing the materials she uses for insulin injections.[14(p 43)]

### What's It Like in the Hospital?*

Among the important things to consider about the hospital care of adolescents is knowing that they are overly concerned about themselves even when they are not sick, and even more so when they are ill. Harsh authority and inconsiderate supervision "turns them off." They will resent restrictions of activity and do not wish to be stripped of their newly attained sense of growing independence. They will be anxious about separation from family and friends. They will feel uncomfortable in unfamiliar situations.

As a countermeasure, visits by peers and family should be encouraged. Peer interaction, which is most intense during adolescence, can be used to advantage.[15(p 213)] Communal meals, group activities arranged by recreational therapists, and weekly meetings of patients led by a social worker or child psychiatrist help hospitalized teenagers in their adjustments. Schowalter and Anyan report the initiation of a hospital ward newspaper in one teenage unit.[15(p 213)]

In addition, it is helpful for staff members just to visit and talk with the patient from time to time.[16(p 47)] Even though communications about medical problems are usually carried out with parents, adolescents want and should have personal discussions with their physicians and nurses.

*This issue is dealt with extensively in Chapter 8.*

## THE AGE OF CONSENT—WHAT IS IT?

Most states prohibit minors from receiving health care without parental consent. Minors are usually considered to be those persons who are under 18 years of age.

However, certain states have already liberalized their laws, and legislation is pending in others. Most health professionals who work with adolescents are happy to see these changes, pointing out that they are merely a formal sanction for what has been going on all along.[2(p 70)] Too many times, minors are in need of health care but are too far away from home for parental consent to be immediately obtained. Some teenagers have strained relationships with their parents and for this reason it would be convenient to have liberalized laws that would provide for waiving parental consent. The concept of "emancipated minor" qualifies some teenagers for being able to make their own decisions about receiving personal health care. Those teenagers who are married, living away from home and contributing toward 50 percent of their support, or are members of the military service do not need parental consent.

At Mount Sinai, as in many other settings, physicians may use their discretion about which patients they will see without parental consent. With medical crises, Dr. Thomas Shaffer stated that at Columbus Children's Hospital the policy is that two physicians must put in writing that an emergency exists and that the minor requires treatment. This allows for a minor's emergency medical treatment. Quoting Dr. Joan E. Morgenthau, "We've been assured that there's never been a national case in which a parent has brought suit against someone for judiciously administering necessary medical care to a minor."[2(p 70)]

## SUMMARY

Adolescence is for most teenagers a health phase of the life cycle. What they look like, how "normal" they are, and what others think of them are common concerns of adolescents in our society. When illness occurs, these concerns are often magnified far out of proportion by the patient.

Several types of health subsystems exist to guide the adolescent in maintaining and attaining a degree of high level wellness, and these have been discussed in this chapter. Understanding the teenage patient and instilling in him a sense of independence, recognition, and respect as an individual are important in establishing a trusting relationship between the patient and the health care professional. Limitations are set to demonstrate concern and afford the temporary dependence that is sometimes necessary. The ideal situation exists when the goals are agreed upon by the health professionals in conjunction with their teenage patients, and these goals are communicated, understood, and implemented by the teenagers themselves, and by their parents and family members.

## REFERENCES

1. Rigg CA, Fisher RC: Some comments on current hospital medical services for adolescents. American Journal of Diseased Child Vol 120, Sept 1970, pp 193–96
2. Pembrook L: Adolescent clinics: a vital step in solving the problems of teenagers. Parent's Magazine, Nov 1972, pp 68–70
3. Blaise Sister Mary: Rationale and planning for an adolescent unit. Supervision Nurse, Sept 1972, p 37
4. Characteristics of an inpatient unit for adolescents. Clin Pediatr, Jan 1973, p 18

5. Blake F et al: Nursing Care of Children. Philadelphia, Lippincott, 1970
6. Hammar SL, Eddy JA: Nursing Care of the Adolescent. New York, Springer, 1966
7. Marlow DR: Textbook of Pediatric Nursing. Philadelphia, Saunders, 1973
8. Cooke RE (ed): The Biologic Basis of Pediatric Practice. New York, McGraw-Hill, 1968
9. Daniel WA Jr: The Adolescent Patient. St Louis, Mosby, 1970
10. Daubenmire MJ et al: Adolescence in the hospital. Nursing Outlook, Sept 1960
11. Conway B: The effect of hospitalization on adolescence. Adolescence 6:77–92, 1971
12. Schindler-Rainman E: Communicating with today's teenagers: an exercise between generations. Children, Nov–Dec 1969
13. American Academy of Pediatrics: Care of Children in Hospitals. Presentation. Evanston, Illinois, 1963
14. Ashburn SS: A study to determine the effects of juvenile diabetes mellitus on the biopsychosocial needs of the thirteen-to-fifteen year old female with consequent nursing care implications. Unpublished Master's Thesis, Ohio State U, 1970
15. Schowalter JE, Anyan WR: Experience on an adolescent in-patient division. American Journal of Diseased Child, Vol 125, Feb 1973
16. Heald FP: An Inpatient Unit for Adolescents. National League for Nursing 1963 Convention, May 14, 1963

## BIBLIOGRAPHY

Association for the Care of Children in Hospitals Newsletter, Issue 18, Sept 1972

Erikson EH: Reflections on the dissent of contemporary youth. Int J Psychoanal 51:11–22, 1970

Hofman AD: Patient-Staff-Parent Interrelationships and the Hospital Setting. Sixth Annual Conference of the Association for the Care of Children in the Hospitals, May 1971, pp 46–53

Services for adolescents. American Journal of Diseased Child, Vol 120, Sept 1970, pp 193–96

# 3

# The Teenage Unwed Mother

ELAINE SCHROEDER

Throughout the past few years a great deal has been written about the problem of illegitimacy in our country. Many of the articles and books have been devoted to a discussion of the problem of illegitimacy within the teenage population. Statistics have been quoted, the predisposing causes of illegitimacy have been explored, possible solutions to the problem have been suggested, and yet very little has been written to guide and help the nurse in her efforts to give comprehensive care to the pregnant, unwed teenager within the health care system.

Contrary to popular opinion, the illegitimacy rate among the teenage population is less than half of all out-of-wedlock pregnancies. Approximately 60 percent of the illegitimate births in our country occur in the over-twenty age group, whereas only 40 percent occur in the group under twenty years of age (Table 1).[1] We often read that the number of illegitimate births has risen, although

Table 1

## MARRIED AND OUT-OF-WEDLOCK LIVE BIRTHS BY AGE OF MOTHER FOR 1965 IN THE U.S.[1](p 8)

| MOTHER'S AGE | MARRIED LIVE BIRTHS | OUT-OF-WEDLOCK LIVE BIRTHS | TOTAL LIVE BIRTHS |
|---|---|---|---|
| Under age 15 | 1,668 | 6,100 | 7,768 |
| Age 15—19 | 467,894 | 123,000 | 590,894 |
| Age 20—24 | 1,246,750 | 90,000 | 1,337,350 |
| Age 25—29 | 888,932 | 36,800 | 925,732 |
| Age 30—34 | 509,776 | 19,600 | 529,376 |
| Age 35 & older | 354,238 | 15,000 | 369,238 |

when viewed in relation to the total increase in the number of births in this country, this change is not as remarkable as it may sound.

Although statistics are important in alerting us to the scope of an existent problem, they can also become misleading. Statistics should not be considered out of their original context, but always viewed within the entire scope of the problem being studied.

When the teenager becomes pregnant out-of-wedlock, she is usually forced to enter three spheres, or areas of service—the social service sphere, the educational sphere, and the health care sphere (Fig. 1). It is important that she receive support and help in each of these three areas, for this support will greatly influence her reaction to her pregnancy and the impact it will have on her future life.

Although the nurse will be providing support to the

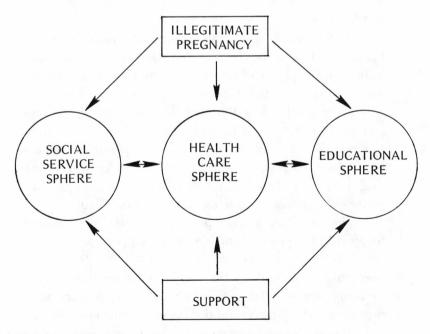

FIG. 1. Three service spheres needed by pregnant unwed teenager.

teenage mother primarily within the health care sphere, she must also be aware that help is needed for the teenager in the two other spheres as well. Social support is often necessary because in our society the unwed mother is often rejected and abandoned by her boyfriend, her family, and her significant peers. As a result, the teenager is often forced to enter the social service sphere to receive guidance, financial help, living arrangements, or adoption services for her baby.

The pregnant teenager needs support in the educational sphere because it has been common practice in many communities for a pregnant girl to be expelled from school as soon as the pregnancy is discovered. Pregnant adolescents who do not continue their education during pregnancy are most likely going to be high school dropouts, and thus ill-prepared to support their families in the world today. The social consequences of an expanding population of poorly educated women who become heads of families can be seen in the rising costs of public welfare and disrupted family relationships.[2]

Within the medical sphere, support should be given in many dimensions. In the past, two factors have seemed to influence the quality of medical care that the unwed teenager has received—the attitudes of the medical profession along with their overburdened medical facilities, and the attitudes and fears of the unwed mother. The features of the medical services offered to unwed mothers are frequently a discouraging factor. Long waits on hard benches in crowded clinics, long distances to travel, frequently changing staff, and lack of privacy have actually made medical care undesirable.[3]

The nurse can be a key person within the medical sphere to provide the physical and emotional support needed by the pregnant teenager. She can also be a coordinator with the two other spheres to see that social and educational support are being provided. To do this the nurse needs to learn all that she can about teenagers and their needs during pregnancy.

Teenage unwed pregnancy presents a unique problem,

and for this reason is most often a cause of great concern. When pregnancy occurs in adolescence, the girl is forced to deal with two maturational crises at the same time—the process of completing her own growth and identity formulation, and the need to adjust to the ongoing process of pregnancy. This can be an almost overwhelming task for the teenage girl.

Adolescence is characterized in our culture as a period of transition—a period when the teenager faces new and frequently different problems. Quite often the adolescent's position in our culture is not clear. Her role is loosely defined at both the entry and transition points of the adolescent period, and this period often presents a set of vague and conflicting roles.[4] During this period of growth, the adolescent struggles for independence, embarks on a frantic search for self-discovery, and wrestles with the acceptance of a new reflection in the mirror as a new body emerges. The concept of body image becomes increasingly important to the developing teenage girl. Moreover, the teenager begins to move from the security of the family group, which is now rejected, to the peer group where acceptance and status are sought.[5]

The central developmental task of adolescence is that of self-definition or identity formation. It is during this period of time in the growth process that the teenager must learn who she is and what she really feels about herself and the world about her. Erikson states that developing a sense of identity carries with it a mastery of the problems of childhood and a general readiness to face, as a potential equal, the challenges of the adult world. Identity depends on becoming counted upon, and on becoming an accountable part of a larger whole.[6]

With these growth tasks of adolescence in mind, it is not difficult to see, then, how pregnancy might influence the developing teenager. The physiologic burdens that the pregnancy imposes upon the growing teenage girl are not to be overlooked, for the period of adolescence itself is marked by many physical changes and rapid growth. A pregnancy at this time imposes more of a physiologic burden upon the teenager than it would upon an adult who has reached physical maturity. It is not surprising, therefore, to note that teenagers seem to have more physical problems throughout their pregnancies than do older mothers. Also, during a period of time when body image is so important to the young girl, it is very difficult for her to adjust to and accept the obvious physical changes of pregnancy.

When the teenage girl becomes pregnant, her struggle for independence becomes more complicated. Very often the girl must give up her desire for independence because of her forced need to become dependent, physically and/or emotionally, upon her family. The task of identity development is also made more difficult. How can a teenager possibly begin to learn to know herself as the young girl that she is, when suddenly she also is forced to learn to know herself as a mother? When the teenager, quite often still a child herself in many ways, must suddenly contemplate the added responsibility of nurturing her own child, problems can easily arise as a result of this role conflict. It is therefore important that the nurse keep in mind the developmental factors of rapid growth, body image, independence, and identity formation as she relates to the pregnant teenager, for many of the behaviors or attitudes that the teenager displays may be influenced by the conflict she is experiencing with these growth tasks.

The nurse needs to consider also the social as well as the physical and emotional influences that might affect the teenager as she progresses through the maternity cycle. Teenagers who become pregnant out-of-wedlock come from all cultures and from all socioeconomic levels. Some are from rural backgrounds, some from urban; some are members of ethnic groups that have had particularly difficult problems because of discrimination; some are "upward mobile" or from wealthy homes, and some are "downward mobile"; some might be from such deviant groups as drug addicts, prostitutes, criminals, or the mentally ill. Even within a culturally homogeneous group, individual personalities and life situations will vary tremendously.[7]

As nurses it is important to remember to take into consideration the social and cultural factors that might influence each pregnant teenager who enters the health care system. It is very easy for the nurse to make the assumption that the attitudes and ethics of each teenager with whom she deals are similar to her own, and this assumption can quickly block her attempts to communicate therapeutically with the pregnant young girl or to provide her with comprehensive supportive care. It is important to remember, for example, that the concepts of illegitimacy, of marriage, or of family, may hold entirely different meanings in various cultures or ethnic groups. As an example, Cahill describes the concept of family life held by the people of the Caribbean and Latin American cultures.[7 (p13)] Within these cultures are several acceptable forms of marriage, the most desirable of which is a legalized union. This is not always feasible, however, because of the economy, because only a few people are authorized to perform marriage, and because of the girl's lack of bargaining power since she may come from a family of weakened structure. As a result, many consensual unions exist. These are not casual relationships, however, and may last for a few months or a lifetime. The offspring of these unions are accepted as legitimate within the culture. If desertion does occur, a maternal family structure results, in that the mother is the only continuing parent. The man is dominant, however, and assumes at least temporary responsibility for the family and readily acknowledges his paternity. The woman does not consider herself to be "illegitimately" pregnant, and hopes eventually to marry. It is easy to see, then, that a girl growing up in such a family structure is likely to have a mother-father role concept which allows her, in turn, to accept such a union for herself—without the stigma which we often attach to this type of family relationship.

This is only one example of the cultural differences that may exist in regard to family life. Each cultural or ethnic group that the nurse encounters may in turn present other unique differences in attitude and life style. It would be of no benefit in establishing a therapeutic relationship for the nurse to impose upon the pregnant teenager her own personal attitudes or cultural beliefs regarding out-of-wedlock pregnancy or family life.

Unfortunately, it is also very easy to begin to classify all unwed mothers into one group. As a result of stereotypic thinking we begin to feel that all unwed teenagers who are pregnant must be alike—that is, they no doubt think alike, they most likely have the same "free" attitudes about sex, they probably do not have a very positive relationship with the boy who got them pregnant, they are no doubt guilty and unhappy about their pregnancy, and they certainly are not going to care much about the baby or be able to provide for it adequately after its birth.

Naturally, generalizations such as these are inappropriate, and can even be dangerous. It is unfair to the pregnant teenager for us to assume anything about her situation or her feelings regarding it. Not *all* teenagers who become pregnant out-of-wedlock have "free" attitudes about sex. Many of them have had a very meaningful relationship with the father of the baby, and plan for this relationship to continue. Some pregnant teenagers are very happy, if not proud, about the fact that they are pregnant, and are actually looking forward to the experience of mothering their child. It is important, then, that each pregnant teenager and each unwed pregnancy be viewed independently and uniquely.

And yet, even though the nurse becomes aware of the social, cultural, and developmental influences upon the pregnant teenager, she may still have her own feelings to deal with. It is important that the nurse recognize her own feelings so she can deal with them openly and realistically, and not allow them to interfere with her ability to support the pregnant teenager. Many nurses admit to reacting with shock or disgust when faced with a teenager who is pregnant out-of-wedlock. It is not uncommon for nurses to want to moralize as they relate to the unwed mother. In an attempt to deal with her own feelings and attitudes, it might be helpful to the nurse to consider what factors are influencing her reactions. What is it that bothers her about an unwed pregnant teenager? Is it the fact that she is quite young, and perhaps does not fully recognize the impact and responsibilities of pregnancy and motherhood? Perhaps the nurse considers the implications that this pregnancy will have for the young girl in terms of loss of personal freedom, interruption or cessation of education, added responsibility, or enforced maturity. She no doubt considers the problems that the teenager's unwed marital status may force upon her in our society, such as social discrimination, financial difficulties, or lack of emotional support. The nurse may think of problems that can occur as a result of the illegitimate pregnancy, such as child neglect and abuse, or future illegitimate pregnancies. Even though the nurse may consider all these facets of illegitimate pregnancy, she must be careful not to project her perception of these problems, or her own reactions to them, upon the teenager, but to discover how the teenager views the pregnancy and what problems, if any, she foresees.

The question that seems to be most frequently asked by both student and graduate nurses is, "How do I talk to the unwed pregnant teenager? What do I say?" The reason that these questions are asked is that nurses tend to put the "unwed" factor first—ahead of the other important factors relating to the mother. The "unwed" factor then becomes a block, because of the nurses' own attitudes, to her abilities to develop a relationship with the mother. It must therefore be kept in mind that the pregnant teenager is first and foremost an individual—a teenager who happens to be pregnant, and who has come into the health care system seeking help. The fact that she is unwed certainly should not be ignored as the nurse plans her care, but should be secondary. The unwed pregnant teenager is not a freak; she is not, in many ways, unlike the married mother, and she displays many of the same needs. She may of course, because of her marital status, have additional needs that can be discovered when working with her. In planning for care, it is important for the nurse to remember that a therapeutic relationship cannot be built overnight. It may take time for the unwed mother to develop trust and confidence in the nurse. Teenagers will often hide their true thoughts and feelings behind a mask of indifference, hostility, unconcern, or boredom. Most often these observable behaviors are an attempt to conceal feelings such as fear, vulnerability, anger, self-consciousness, or depression.

As the nurse begins to develop her plan of care for the pregnant teenager, one of the best ways to determine what needs should be met is to ask the teenager what she feels her needs are in relation to her pregnancy. As nurses, it is easy for us to project our perception of the teenager's needs into our care, when in reality the teenager may not see these as being her needs at all.

In a research study conducted by the author,[8] it was found that unwed pregnant teenagers are very much aware of their physical, emotional, social, and intellectual needs throughout the maternity cycle. These mothers also have very specific ideas regarding the type of help and support that they feel would be beneficial to them. If the nurse consults with the pregnant teenager as she plans her care, the teenager is given the opportunity to share her ideas and feelings regarding her own needs, is made to feel that she has an important part in planning her care and, together, the nurse and teenager can work toward a common goal.

The broad goal for the nurse who is helping the pregnant teenager should be that of helping her to emerge from the experience with as positive an image of herself as a person as her circumstances and personality will permit.[9] Good maternity care for the unwed mother should be expanded and planned to end with an emotionally healthy young woman who is prepared to return to her life routines nurtured by her childbirth experience. The nurse can work towards this goal by being ready whenever possible to deemphasize the unmarried, socially deviant aspects of her experience, and accentuate its normal, healthy components.

As the nurse strives to meet this goal, she will be providing care for the unwed mother in many different ways—physically, emotionally, socially, and educationally. The teenager most frequently views her physical needs as being rather minimal during pregnancy,[8] and the actual physical care that the nurse provides during this time is also usually minimal. The primary function of the nurse should be that of interpreter to the teenager. Any physical care that the teenager does receive should be discussed and explained. For example, the reasons for and the findings of abdominal and vaginal examinations should be explained. A discussion of the status of the baby and his state of growth and development will be very meaningful to the pregnant teenager if she is planning to keep her baby. The reasons for monitoring her weight gain and checking her urine should be explained. The process of labor should be discussed with her, both prior to its onset and during the intrapartal period. The process of involution should be explained during the postpartal period.

Teenagers are often not highly motivated, or are very frightened about coming for routine medical care. There can be many reasons for these attitudes or fears regarding medical supervision, and many of these might be justified. Reasons might include such factors as embarrassment, a wish to hide the pregnancy, fear of what will take place during the examination, transportation problems, long waits in crowded waiting rooms, changing staff, lack of privacy, or a total lack of understanding as to why medical supervision is important during pregnancy. If the nurse will take the time to explain and interpret what is taking place, the pregnant teenager will be made to feel more that she is a participant in her medical care, will understand why supervision is important, and may become more motivated and willing to come for care regularly. The nurse's attitude and interest can often be the deciding factor in whether the teenager will return.

During labor the teenager desires physical support from the nurse in the way of pain relief, continued explanation of what is taking place, patience, sympathetic understanding, and most of all, the physical presence of the nurse—needs which are common to any mother during this period of time, regardless of her marital status. It is important that the nurse recognize the need for the teenager to have with her during labor the person that she trusts and feels will be most helpful to her—whether this be her boyfriend, one of her parents, another family member, or a friend.

In contrast to the physical support of the unwed teenager during her pregnancy, the area of emotional support is much more difficult and challenging. It is also in this area that the pregnant teenager expresses many of her needs.[8] Unwed pregnant teenagers are often eager to talk about their problems, concerns, or feelings regarding their pregnancy, if the nurse will only take the time to allow her to talk, show interest and concern, and listen. Because of her feelings of inadequacy, this area of supportive care is often neglected by the nurse, or passed on to someone else, when in reality it is the nurse who often has the best opportunity to form a trusting relationship with the teenager. Emotional support is important during all periods of the maternity cycle. Through her understanding of crisis, its effect on an individual, and the principles involved in crisis intervention, the nurse can provide a great deal of reassurance to the young expectant mother.

The nurse also can provide support to the teenager in regard to the social influences which might be affecting her, by making an effort to discover what these influences are. A social history collected by the nurse should be an important part in the planning of care for each mother. For example, it is of no benefit to discuss diet with the teenager without first finding out what foods her family enjoys, what foods they can afford, and what influence cultural habits may have upon their dietary regimen. Also, the relationship of the father of the baby to the pregnant teenager is an important social influence upon her, but most frequently he is either ignored or totally forgotten. The teenager very often would like to discuss her feelings about the father of the baby—whether her feelings are positive as a result of the boyfriend being very supportive of her, or whether they are negative as a result of the boyfriend having deserted her.

If there is a decision to be made about whether to keep the baby or give the baby up for adoption, the nurse can also provide support in this area. This decision would be a difficult one for any mother, let alone a mother who is very young. The most effective approach at this time is to allow the teenager to verbalize her feelings and to help her to weigh the advantages and disadvantages of either choice. The nurse may be able to help the teenager to see what effect either of the decisions might have upon all of the people involved. Although she can help the teenager to think through the problem, and to weigh various factors in making her decision, the nurse should never give her personal opinions or give advice to the teenager regarding this decision. The final decision must be that of the teenager and her family.

The need most frequently expressed by pregnant unwed teenagers is that of education regarding their childbirth experience.[8] Even though teenage mothers may appear to be disinterested or unconcerned, they really do want to learn and to be informed. Teenagers often are merely embarrassed to admit they do not know something, or are afraid to take the time of the doctor or nurse. Nurses therefore should not let themselves be deceived by the outward behaviors they observe. Teenage mothers want to know all about their diet, the changing signs and symptoms of pregnancy, fetal growth and development, signs of labor, the process of labor and delivery, procedures they will encounter, how they can help themselves during labor, postpartal care, infant care, and birth control. Teaching should be done continuously by the nurse no matter in what phase of the maternity cycle she comes in contact with the teenage mother.

When giving information to the teenager several factors should be considered. It is important that information be given at both the intellectual and emotional level of the teenager. Facts should be presented simply and the nurse should verify the teenager's understanding of what she has heard, by giving her an opportunity to repeat the information or to ask questions. Teaching will be much more effective if the nurse will discover the area of interest that is of present concern to the teenager. For example, providing a great deal of information to the teenager about fetal growth and development will be of little value if at that point in time her anxieties and concerns are related to the process of labor. Instruction need not be presented in a rigid or chronologic sequence. If the teenager's concerns at the present time relate to the birth process—even though this process may still be some distance off—this is the information that should be given. Other important information can then be given at a later time—when the teenager is better able to accept it.

It is also important to be cautious about feeding information to the teenager without first having discussed the subject with her, finding her present level of understanding, and what questions she may have. When teaching is undertaken as a one-way process, that is, the nurse merely giving the information, this discourages the teenager from expressing such things as "wive's tales" she may have heard, questions she wishes to ask, or anxieties that she may have. By merely having information fed to her, the teenager will be made to feel that her questions or concerns are probably "silly" or "stupid." Teaching is more effective when it becomes a two-way interchange between nurse and teenager.

Teaching can be carried out on an informal one-to-one basis, or more formally in group sessions. If the time and scheduling factor is a problem, a great deal of teaching can be performed by the nurse while she is working with the teenager in other ways. For example, the nurse can furnish information about diet while she is weighing the teenager and taking her blood pressure. While the nurse is preparing the teenager to be examined by the doctor, she can discuss with her the symptoms of pregnancy that she is experiencing, can explain the reasons for them, and can inform her about what she might expect in the future. Throughout labor the nurse can be continually teaching while she is doing such other procedures as checking the vital signs, giving the enema, preparing the perineal area, or examining the teenager to determine her progress in labor.

The postpartal period provides an excellent opportunity for instruction, for at this time the teenage mother is a captive audience. Teaching should therefore be one of the primary functions of the nurse working in the postpartal area. Not only will information about herself and the involutional process be important to her, but the teenager will want to know a great deal about how to care for her baby. These young mothers should be taught about the normal characteristics of the newborn, how to feed, hold, and burp the baby, how to bathe the baby, and what might be expected of the baby when they get home. Information about various methods of birth control should be explained and discussed with the teenager prior to her discharge from the hospital. The importance of continued medical supervision should also be explained to her. The role of educational support, then, is an enormously important one for the nurse who is working with the teenage mother and should never for a moment be minimized.

The need for total comprehensive support of the

teenage unwed mother is a great one. This need can be met more easily by the nurse if she will take into consideration the developmental tasks of adolescence that may influence the teenager and the social and cultural factors that are involved. The nurse must learn to examine her own feelings and attitudes and avoid stereotypic thinking. Support for the pregnant teenager should be given physically, emotionally, socially, and educationally throughout the maternity cycle. The challenge to the nurse is unlimited, and the results of her efforts can be vastly rewarding.

## REFERENCES

1. Osofsky HJ: The Pregnant Teenager. Springfield, Ill, Charles C Thomas, 1968, p 4
2. McMurray G: Continuing education for teenage parents. Nurs Outlook 17:12, Dec 1969, p 66
3. Bernstein R: Gaps in services to unmarried mothers. Children, March–April 1965, p 49
4. Garrison KC: Psychology of Adolescence. Englewood Cliffs, NJ, Prentice-Hall, 1965, p 18
5. Clark A: The crisis of adolescent unwed motherhood. Am J Nurs 67:7, July 1967, p 1465
6. Erikson EH: Identity: Youth and Crisis. New York, Norton, 1968, p 128
7. Cahill ID: Facts and fallacies concerning pregnancy out of wedlock. In Jeffries JE (ed): The Adolescent Unwed Mother. Ross Round-table on Maternal and Child Nursing, Ross Laboratories, Columbus, Ohio, 1965, p 12
8. Schroeder E: A descriptive study of the subjective needs of of the unwed mother throughout the maternity cycle. Unpublished thesis, Ohio State U, 1972
9. Bernstein R: Are we still stereotyping the unwed mother? Social Work 5:3, 1960, p 100

## BIBLIOGRAPHY

Aguilera DC, Messick JM, Farrel MS: Crisis Intervention: Theory and Methodology. St Louis, Mosby, 1970
Bernstein R: Are we still stereotyping the unwed mother? Social Work 5:3, 1960, p 100
——————— : Gaps in services to unmarried mothers. Children, Mar–April 1965, p 49

Cahill ID: Facts and fallacies concerning pregnancy out of wedlock. In Jeffries JE (ed): The Adolescent Unwed Mother. Ross Roundtable on Maternal and Child Nursing, Ross Laboratories, Columbus, Ohio, 1965, p 12

Cassidy JT: Teenagers in a family planning clinic. Nurs Outlook 18:11, Nov 1970, p 30

Clark A: The crisis of adolescent unwed motherhood. Am J Nurs 67:7, July 1967, p 1465

Erikson EH: Identity: Youth and Crisis. New York, Norton, 1968

Garrison KC: Psychology of Adolescence. Englewood Cliffs, NJ, Prentice-hall, 1965

Malo-Juvera D: What pregnant teenagers know about sex. Nurs Outlook 18:11, Nov 1970, p 32

McMurray G: Continuing education for teenage parents. Nurs Outlook 17:12, Dec 1969, p 66

Naugle EN: Nurse make it well. Nurs Outlook 18:11, Nov 1970

Osofsky HJ: The Pregnant Teenager. Springfield, Ill, Charles C Thomas, 1968

Pannor R: The forgotten man. Nurs Outlook 18:11, Nov 1970, p 41

Parad HJ (ed): Crisis Intervention: Selected Readings. New York, Family Service Association of America, 1970, p 36

Schroeder E: A descriptive study of the subjective needs of the unwed mother throughout the maternity cycle. Unpublished Thesis, Ohio State U, 1972

# 4

# The School - Its Relationship to Health Services

NANCY M. BRUCE AND ALICE E. DAWSON

The school plays a major role in health services for the adolescent. In accord with its major responsibility for enhancing the young person's potential and providing him with the capacities to function in an adult society, the school must recognize and be prepared to provide for his health care needs. Likewise, the health care facility must seek to understand and appreciate the impact of the school on the life circumstances of the teenager. To disregard or minimize the school's role is to fail to understand the teenager as a total being.

This chapter is devoted to an examination of the more common physical and emotional problems of adolescents, the respective roles of the school and the health care facility in recognizing these, and the interrelationship of both facilities in their management.

## CONSULTATION AND COLLABORATION

The school is a primary referral resource as well as a vital supportive agency. When one considers the vast percentage of time the teenager spends in school or in educational endeavors, this fact becomes strikingly obvious. To the health care facility dealing with adolescents this is perhaps made even more obvious by the upswing of referrals during the school year. Nearly any hospital or clinic serving youth will report an increase in requests for service that coincides with the opening of school.

An increase in the understanding of the educational system should then provide a vehicle for offering enhanced and more comprehensive adolescent health services. Perhaps cooperative efforts with the school might be divided into two categories by viewing the school as (1) a referral resource, (2) a collaborator.

### The School as a Referral Resource

Referrals emanate from the school and school personnel in many forms. Attempts to explore and understand the source and manner of these referrals can lead to an appreciation of the perceptive elements within the school for identification of problems.

Perhaps to understand these elements one might begin by identifying school personnel who are likely to recognize problems and bring them to the attention of a health service agency. The school nurse is the primary referral resource, but counselors, administrators, and visiting teachers or school social workers are also active in identifying problems and seeking diagnostic assessments or follow-up.

## THE SCHOOL NURSE

The *school nurse* tends to be a standard position in most high schools and junior highs in the United States. Although not always a full-time staff member, the nurse is generally available to the school for routine health care evaluation and follow-up. For school nurses involved with adolescents, this role is often expanded to include evaluation and follow-up for mental health problems as well. Perhaps because of her identification with the medical profession the school nurse often looks first to the health care facility for the evaluation of both health and mental health types of problems.

## THE ADMINISTRATOR

School administrators in the junior high and high school are generally identified as the principal, assistant principal, and dean of students. All three positions are usually held by personnel with several years of teaching experience as well as a master's degree in secondary school administration. Although direct pupil contact is usually greater with both the dean of students and assistant principal, all school administrators spend, whether by choice or not, an inordinate amount of time with the management of adolescent health as well as mental health problems.

## THE COUNSELOR

The counselor is now a standard position in most secondary schools but the role varies according to the individual as well as the setting. Most counselors are teacher trained, many with actual teaching experience that personally acquaints them with classroom problems. Standard training for the counselor position is then a master's degree in guidance and counseling within a college of education. Depending on the college program as well as the interests of the individual pursuing the degree, emphasis can be placed on either academic or personal counseling techniques. Likewise, dependent on the emphasis in the individual secondary school or guidance department, an emphasis is placed on one of these two areas.

THE VISITING TEACHER OR SCHOOL SOCIAL WORKER

The roles of the visiting teacher or school social worker are alike for the most part in that both have multifaceted roles ranging from a primary focus on school absenteeism to mental health consultation with other school personnel. In most states the school social worker—visiting teacher possesses a two-year master's degree in social work; in others the worker holds an education degree. Regardless of their specific roles these personnel generally are reasonably well known by the faculty and student body. In many instances if the school social worker does not know a problem student directly, he does have indirect knowledge of any difficulties.

Most school referrals to a health care facility are initiated directly by the personnel named, and the telephone call or letter requesting service usually indicates a desire for a complete evaluation. These may or may not be accompanied by background information on the patient.

Whether or not background information does accompany the referral, the first step to be taken by the health care professional should be to contact the referring agent. Although the intake person must maintain a focus on the services that his institution is equipped to provide, this must not overshadow a respect for what the referring agent presents as the complaint. In other words, start with the complaint as it is seen by the school and then proceed to develop an understanding of the problem in terms of your respective agency's capacity for servicing it.

Key information might focus first on a description of the problem and what has precipitated the referral, to an understanding of its duration, and any previous attempts at service. Next, but equally as important, is an understanding and appreciation for the involvement of the parent or guardian and the teenager in the request for help.

Based on the information compiled, a decision can be made on whether to accept the case in terms of the institution's capacity for meeting the need. Sometimes another facility better equipped to meet the need is indicated. It is our feeling that the intake professional's responsibility does not end with evaluating his institution's capacity for handling the problem or even with scheduling a diagnostic assessment. If an appropriate resource is available within the community, his guiding the school referral agent to that resource is as valuable as the provision of service itself. Most communities have developed a directory of social service and health care agencies that should facilitate this process.

Although the preceding discussion seems to ignore the parent or child himself within the referral process, they are by no means meant to be excluded. For the most part, however, their request for service will have been based on previous consultation with one of the key school personnel. Certainly direct contact by them is to be encouraged, and in those instances in which the school referring agent has not discussed the request for service with the student and/or family, such discussion should be discreetly urged. In the same vein, any parent who requests service for his teenage son or daughter should likewise be encouraged to permit consultation with the school.

## The School as Collaborator

Perhaps this is one of the most valuable, yet one of the most disregarded services that the school has the capacity to offer.

Whether the adolescent has come to the health care facility as a school referral or of his own accord, his health care needs will likely pervade the educational spheres of his life. Consequently, whether the need is for follow-up of a physical or mental health nature, the school personnel are a valuable professional resource to the health care agency.

In terms of the student's health care needs, the school nurse should probably be the resource person to involve. She not only has the professional training to understand the young person's medical problems and deal with his needs for care, but she has the necessary expertise to interpret them to staff members who might be involved. For the medical or allied medical professional, the school nurse can and usually is eager to act as liaison agent.

In terms of the student's mental health needs, any or all of the school personnel named are valuable resources for many follow-up requirements. Although the health professional should be able to offer knowledge and clarification on specific problems referred, his professional maturity is enhanced by his ability to recognize the areas in which school personnel might utilize their expertise. At the same time it is important that he perceive overdependence on the part of the school personnel who might otherwise be effective collaborators.

Enlistment of the services of the school can be done personally and/or by letter. My preference places an emphasis on the former with a suggestion that staff conferences either at school or health care facility are usually enlightening experiences for both agencies. It might be important to note as well that often lasting relationships develop from such individual case conferences. Most school personnel can be elicited as collaborators by a simple invitation, but many, in particular those who may not have experienced such activity, may require much support and a show of appreciation to incorporate this as a part of their role.

## COMMON PHYSICAL DISORDERS

### Psychophysiologic Problems

Physical symptomatology is often the means for an adolescent to express stress. Symptoms may include stomachaches, headaches, or vague feelings of malaise, but whatever the symptom, it should be viewed as a possible means of his gaining admission to some sort of support system.

The student may appear repeatedly at the school nurse's office or visit the health care facility with a recital of complaints. Of course, a medical evaluation should be undertaken, but the importance of the symptomatology to the teenager should be explored regardless of the medical findings. It might be expected that this will commonly uncover important information. The teenager, given a chance to respond to the question, "Is anything bothering you?" may have been waiting to open the subject for discussion, and an atmosphere of acceptance and support is essential to helping him. Often the reassurance of a health care professional that no physical reason can be found for the complaint will be an important factor in releasing the adolescent to discuss his other concerns.

The teenager who learns that he can get attention and discuss problems without resorting to physical complaints is developing important skills in coping with his own problems. School personnel can reinforce this kind of mature response through daily contacts with the adolescent.

Frequently the kinds of symptoms presented mask serious emotional or family problems. If the family is unreceptive or cannot respond, the adolescent may have few people to turn to to discuss intimacies. Particularly if a supportive peer group is not available to him, or their concern and sympathy not enough, the youth may have need of institutional services that he can use without involving parental consent. Both the school and the health care facility are sources available to him that he can use as acceptable routes for getting help. It is not uncommon that a referral for family therapy might result from a fifteen-year-old's having told a school nurse about his headaches.

> Susan, age 14, made extensive visits to the nurse's office at school with severe, debilitating headaches. She would frequently have to leave school because of these, but would usually return the following morning. She was an intelligent, but very quiet and sensitive girl who appeared to be chronically anxious and fearful. Her school grades were adequate but not exceptional. The nurse recommended that she be examined by a physician, and after many delays, finally had to insist to the student's mother that this be done. A thorough medical evaluation revealed no apparent physical basis for the headaches; however, an extensive interview with Susan revealed significant problems. It was found that an older uncle living with the family had been having sexual relations with Susan for some time. On the strong recommendations of the physician, Susan was moved to a sister's home. Once out of the home, Susan's headaches ceased dramatically. She has continued intermittent sharing of feelings with the school nurse and is concurrently followed in our adolescent clinic.

Adolescence is a highly emotional time, and turbulent feelings may intensify symptomatology so severely that the accepted axiom, "the gravity of the symptoms parallels the gravity of the disease" may not be of much value when applied to the adolescent.[1] Hyperventilation episodes or fainting illustrate this, and can be a dramatic and disturbing condition to be dealt with by both school and medical facility. A calm response to such episodes helps to alleviate the adolescent's acute anxiety which is a precipitating factor, but anxious, alarmed adults often increase his panic and fears. Secondary gain, and thus repeated episodes, often result. It is important for these adolescents that they have the opportunity, within the school setting, to discuss their anxieties rather than be overcome by them. The opportunity to be able to talk with a counselor, nurse, or teacher when a crisis looms is vital. Consultation and follow-up care can be offered by the health care facility, but the ongoing management can most effectively be done at school.

An interesting situation of "contagious hyperventilation" which came to the attention of our adolescent clinic illustrates some of the problems that schools and hospitals face in diagnosing and treating this kind of disorder. Three girls, all moderately retarded and all from the same class at school, appeared during a one-month period with relatively similar symptoms of dizziness, stomachache, and fainting spells in school. Harriet, age 14, had been followed in our clinic for some time for "passing out" as often as three times per week. A complete physical evaluation, including EEG, revealed no medical basis for the problem. Harriet did indicate, however, that she was very unhappy with her placement in the "dummies" class. She had been brought to the Emergency Room three times subsequent to our initial contact, usually having been sent there from school. As episodes continued, the school staff became extremely concerned and finally excluded her from class until a medical statement could be secured.

These events occurred close to the time that Mary, the second girl in this trio, came to the clinic. Mary, age 15, had been in the special education class with Harriet for a year. She was brought to our clinic for a medical evaluation of stomach pain, headaches, and "passing out" spells. For several months she had had these symptoms, which she and her family attributed to the smell of paint in the newly painted school room. Mary's symptoms had seemed to develop in the morning at school. Preliminary medical evaluation revealed no physical basis for the condition. A diagnosis of hyperventilation syndrome was made. Further exploration with her, however, revealed that Mary was unhappy at home, where her parents were quite rigid and punitive. She saw school as unsatisfying and was considering dropping out.

The day after Mary was seen, Virginia, age 14, came to the clinic for medical evaluation of the fainting spell that she had had in class that day. Virginia presented as an obese, quiet girl who had a paralytic right foot as the result of childhood polio. She stated in clinic that she had passed out once every day the past week. These spells had usually occurred at the lunch hour, and had never occurred outside of school. The school nurse reported that during these experiences Virginia had become tearful and distraught. A medical evaluation revealed no physical basis for her symptoms, but it was learned that she was often ridiculed by the other students—particularly during lunch hour. A tentative diagnosis of anxiety reaction, with fainting spells due to hyperventilation, was made.

Although these three girls were seen by different physicians, and had not been referred in a group, the school, when contacted, indicated concern and frustration with their common problem. Thus, a joint meeting was planned with our staff and several representatives from the school. At this meeting medical information was shared and reassurance given school personnel that the girls were not physically ill. It was conveyed that with appropriate handling the common problems could probably be resolved within the school setting. A discussion of the secondary gains that the girls might be getting from these episodes was of most help to the school staff. They, for instance, had not been aware that emergency squad runs to the hospital perhaps intensified the problem, reinforcing the girls' strong need for attention and special treatment. The school teachers and nurses were given specific instructions on handling further attacks with a focus on the girls' individual needs. For instance, it was determined that the lunch room was too disturbing to Virginia, and arrangements were made for her to eat in a more quiet classroom. School personnel were assured that the girls could be followed medically as well as concurrently by our clinic social worker. Later contacts with the school revealed a fairly dramatic cessation of symptoms. At the end of two weeks there had been no further "passing out" incidents, and the more comfortable and individualized approaches by the school and our clinic have helped to sustain this.

## Chronic Diseases

Adolescents with chronic diseases present special problems to both the school and health care facility. All teenagers have to adjust to the changes in their bodies but the task of the chronically ill teenager is much greater. At the same time that he is adjusting to the "differentness" of adolescence, he is also adjusting his own to "differentness" from peers. These are contradictory and very frustrating tasks for him. The school and health care facility can work cooperatively to assist both the adolescent and his family toward achieving for him as reasonable an academic, social, and physical adjustment as possible. The school can promote health expectations, and the health care facility can encourage educational pursuits.

### DIABETES

Diabetes is one of the more common chronic illnesses among youth. Particularly as there are no visible manifestations of the disease, the adjustment problems may be overlooked or taken for granted. But to the diabetic adolescent, the fear of differentness is paramount, and many are likely to risk endangering their health to avoid revealing a disability.

The responsiveness of the school with a matter-of-fact acceptance of his needs can greatly enhance the adolescent's adjustment. The school nurse, for example, can discreetly provide the student with a private place for injecting his insulin and testing his urine. In addition, she can eliminate exaggerated responses from staff by providing them with basic medical information about the disease. Unnecessary restrictions of the teenager's activity should be avoided at all costs. Dr. Charles Swift, who completed a pilot study of juvenile diabetics from a psychologic and social point of view, reported his feeling that much ignorance continues to exist in relation to diabetes. He cited an instance in which a fifteen-year-old diabetic girl had been encouraged to engage a tutor because her teachers felt she might "pass out" in school.[2]

Management of the disease should be handled jointly by the teenager and his physician, but ongoing exchanges of information with the school can eliminate unnecessary crises and dispel concerns of staff. For the most part, parents should prove responsive to such an exchange as even the best regulated students are likely to rebel once in awhile and may need the assistance of a calm, well-informed school staff, as evinced by the following:

John W., age 16, was admitted to the hospital when he had become acutely ill after having stopped taking his insulin. When interviewed he presented as bitter and profoundly depressed that he should be burdened with the disease of diabetes. What he, in fact, had been trying to do was to challenge his disease. This was an exaggerated instance of denial, but many diabetics at one time or another have a need to challenge the disease in the belief it will disappear. A resolution of the disappointment can follow. In John's case, the need to challenge his disease had been provoked by a feeling that at school he was seen as weaker and less adequate than other boys. According to John, "I want any guy my size to feel free to fight, not pity me."

He refused follow-up counseling at the hospital even though he had resolved the need to take the insulin. There was another resource, however, and when the school counselor's name, Mr. Foster, was mentioned, John responded positively. He admitted that he had feelings he wanted to share yet resented coming to a medical facility. Mr. Foster responded positively, and expressed a desire for ongoing consultation with the hospital.

SICKLE CELL ANEMIA

Recent educational campaigns have greatly increased the public's awareness of sickle cell anemia. However, large segments of the population still do not clearly understand the difference between sickle cell anemia and sickle cell trait. Nor do they understand some of the problems in daily living that confront an adolescent with the disease. The school, however, plays an extremely important role in the health care of these youth.

A look at the kinds of problems faced by a teenager with sickle cell anemia will show clearly why school personnel are so important. The youngster must visit the doctor and/or hospital frequently; he is likely to have frequent crises which may keep him out of school for weeks or more at a time; he must take special medication. The youth with sickle cell anemia may have strong feelings of inferiority because of his disease, and because he may be small and slender for his age. Certainly at times he must resent the restriction of activities and the need to protect against infections that might precipitate crises.[3]

The school staff aware of these problems must take responsibility for helping the adolescent and his family plan school life accordingly. School activities are important for, as with any adolescent, the youngster should be encouraged to maintain strong, active ties with his peer group. The teenager with sickle cell anemia may need some encouragement, however, to join appropriate activities that are satisfying but not too fatiguing for him. Special talents such as drama, music, and managerial skills may need to be uncovered and encouraged in the adolescent who cannot be permitted to engage in sports. Teachers need to familiarize themselves with the signs of a crisis so that they can encourage the adolescent to handle it appropriately. The staff certainly can be helpful in arranging for continuing education should the teenager miss too many days of school because of crises. Coordination of medical records between health care facility and school is extremely important, and transfers to new schools should involve maintenance of similar clear lines of communication.

> Martha K., age 15, had been hospitalized 45 times for sickle cell crises and related complications. She had a good understanding of her disease and the limitations that it imposed upon her, but she had never been able to discuss this freely with school personnel. Her mother, a quiet, unsophisticated woman, from a rural background with little education, did not have the ability to assist Martha in approaching school or public health personnel. Her mother, in fact, relied on Martha to help the family maneuver through the mass of community resources involved in their situation. Martha developed a fairly severe problem with leg ulcers, not an uncommon complication of sickle cell anemia. The ulcers were difficult to treat, and the healing process was slow. The school personnel were sympathetic to Martha's medical problem but knew little about sickle cell anemia. They became concerned that the leg ulcers might indicate a contagious condition and asked Martha's mother to keep her out of school.

> Martha's physician recognized the problem, and asked a social worker to arrange a joint conference between school personnel and health care professionals. At that conference Martha's condition was thoroughly discussed, symptoms of crises and complications of leg ulcers were explained, and educational plans were made for anticipated absences. Martha was immediately readmitted to school. The conference had paved the way for future contacts between the medical facility and school. Indeed the physician, social worker, and nurse were invited to speak to a teacher's in-service training workshop on chronic health problems such as sickle cell anemia.

## THE HANDICAPPED STUDENT

Health problems related to school are likewise related to various categories of handicapped adolescents in the population. Such categories might be divided according to some of the special services of the public school system. Most school systems provide or arrange special services for the following categories of handicapped youth at the secondary level: (1) the physically handicapped, (2) the mentally retarded, (3) the emotionally disturbed.

Although each category as well as each teenager within the category presents a unique and challenging set of symptoms and behaviors, it seems apparent to me that the emotional, mental, and physical health needs of these youth must be seen as inseparable in terms of a total school-health focus. These teenagers present unique and challenging kinds of complaints that need to be understood by the medical professional who wishes to treat them—and who needs to cooperate with the school in doing so.

## The Physically Handicapped Teenager

Physically handicapped teenagers most likely to come to the attention of the health care facility and school are: the visually handicapped, deaf or hard of hearing, and orthopedically handicapped. The adolescent years are particularly tender ones for youth with physical handicaps because of their need to move more toward independent functioning and identification with peer group. Efforts of both are hampered by the youth's need to monitor his condition as well as to accept his obvious differences. His educational plans must therefore not be dominated by any emphasis of the defect—rather by an analysis of his capabilities to function within the system.

It is obvious that every member of the school faculty involved with these students should be familiar with whatever medical services are being offered them, and I would see it as a responsibility of the health care professional to offer faculty members any assistance needed. If the goal is for the teacher and the school staff to share responsibility for noticing any deviations in the student's health, overtures to them in the form of providing information about what to look for should bring about necessary cooperation. The faculty's regular observation of the student's health or mental health status can be one of the most valuable tools in maintaining regular health care.

A report of health care findings and recommendations should be in writing and should constitute a part of the youth's permanent record. Whether the school nurse is custodian of the records or they are a part of his accumulative file, their contents should be accessible to the student's teacher and to the general staff. In many cases a written report is not sufficient and a conference between staff members and medical facility can lead to more effective sharing of ideas. Although there are advantages to having such a conference at the health care facility, the school as a setting will permit the health care worker to acquaint himself with the facilities available. The student should benefit from dual efforts of school personnel who stress the educational aspects of his life and medical consultants who evaluate the setting in terms of health aspects.

Another dual responsibility of the school and health care professional is that of interpreting to parents the student's needs in dealing with their anxieties about his progress. For the normal adolescent this period of independent strivings is particularly anxiety-provoking to parents; their son or daughter slips from their grasp and moves toward identification with the values of his peer group. For parents of a disabled adolescent this process can be complicated by a history of the youth's more dependent status and by the condition of any assumed guilt the parents have yet to resolve.

The type of teamwork required for dealing with the family of a handicapped adolescent requires the closest of cooperation between the health care worker and the school as the family must not be confused by differing opinions.[4] Sustained communication between the two, along with a developed mutual appreciation for the area of expertise of each, will eliminate the necessity for rigidly limiting the area that each will discuss.

Despite the teamwork developed, the right of the teenager and his family to plan for educational and health follow-up must be held in the highest regard. This will be insured if the cooperation starts with the sanction and written permission of the parents. It will never be the responsibility of the professionals involved to impose opinions on the family, even if they feel the members are not choosing wisely. In line with this, the health professional dealing with the adolescent must insist in upholding the youth's dignity and responsibility for making decisions that affect his life. Both parent and teenager can inadvertently abdicate these responsibilities in view of what they see as the professional's expertise and competence for guiding them. This can be guarded against as the health care worker continuously engages in self-evaluation to differentiate his role of expert and counselor.

John, age 13, was referred to our adolescent clinic for adjustment difficulties related to a visual handicap. An otherwise attractive child with above average intelligence, John had disrupted school and family life by temper outbursts, many associated with attempts to deny his handicap. The parents had vacillated between being overprotective and allowing inappropriate liberties. In response to wishing to protect him, the parents had sent him to a school for the blind rather than explore public school programs for the visually handicapped. There, John's interactions had been made up primarily of confrontation with school authorities and peers; their emphasis was on his acceptance of his blindness—his on the fact that he was not blind.

The initial service offered by our staff was clarification of the school problems. A conference with the school psychologist revealed that John, in fact, could probably function in public school, but behavior difficulties had, in his opinion, warranted against this. Lack of staff had made it difficult to provide sufficient counseling to assist the boy in overcoming his adjustment problems. Our agency thus agreed to offer that counseling and arrange, if possible, for transfer to public school once some of the problems began to be resolved. John was later enrolled in the public school program for the visually handicapped, and regular consultation between the resource teacher and our agency has proven to support adequate adjustment. In initiating the cooperation of the new school, the patient's psychosocial and medical records were made available—in response, reports of his progress forwarded to us.

## The Mentally Retarded

School referrals of retarded adolescents represent a large portion of the population in any medical care facility. Both the adolescent's emotional and medical care needs may have presented perpetual confusion to the school. An appreciation of the school's concerns can be developed immediately as the medical care professional is able to focus on his own feelings regarding the management of care.

The quality of teaching and attitudes toward retarded teenagers will vary widely from school to school, but, in general, special classes and equipment are either overcrowded or not readily available. In addition, funding is a perpetual problem, and teachers often feel defeated. Thus a major responsibility of the health care professional will be in terms of collaboration with the school toward location of and referral to resources, carrying out recommendations for treatment, and dealing with parents. Such an assumption of responsibility will greatly encourage the school in working with the adolescent.

Although not unexpected, often the school's perception of problems will vary from that of the parents. A recent study at the adolescent clinic in Seattle, Washington, showed a striking discrepancy between parental and professional assessment of behavior problems, particularly those related to "immaturity and dependency."[5] School personnel noted as problematic the students' failure to develop sufficient self-help skills while parents, more content to foster dependency, were found to be more complacent about the issue.

Based on these findings, I would think a major responsibility of the health care facility treating mentally retarded adolescents first would be to clarify the request for service by exploring the school's and the parents' perceptions of the problem. Second, an attempt to resolve any apparent differences should result in more effective service to the teenager. With regard to the issue of parents fostering their child's dependency, the health care professional is in a position to work more effectively with the parents toward a goal of more separate and individualized functioning for the adolescent, as shown in the following:

Teresa A., age 13, was brought to adolescent clinic by her mother to "find out if she was retarded." According to the mother, the patient was showing great frustration with school, and their family was under pressure from the administration to correct Teresa's behavior. The mother stated that she had had little interpretation regarding Teresa's intellectual ability or the education services being offered her.

Our agency found the school most cooperative in providing information concerning Teresa's previous intellectual evaluation. They were also most interested and understanding about her mother's reported failure to comprehend Teresa's intellectual limitations. Data obtained from school and Teresa's medical history was used in exploring her mother's concerns. Additional evaluation was arranged at a University research center for the mentally retarded. This information was conveyed to the school as well as interpreted to the mother. Subsequently a conference was called at the school; present were Teresa's teachers, the school nurse, the principal, one of our resident physicians, a clinic social worker, and Teresa's mother. Professional recommendations regarding Teresa's intellectual deficiencies and behavior problems were shared with one another and with Mrs. A. while mutual concerns were discussed. A pattern in terms of open communication seemed to have been established.

The Seattle study also affirmed what might have been assumed would be an area of concern shared by parents and school personnel alike.[5] Sexual behavior of the mentally retarded adolescent is in general an issue that provokes anxiety and feelings of relative helplessness in parents and professionals. Complaints regarding male retardates most frequently seem to be involved with exhibitionism and masturbation. With girls, complaints generally seem to relate to menstrual hygiene, risk of pregnancy, and masturbation.

For many of the same reasons that the retardate has been

shielded from other developmental activities, he is likely to
have been neglected in his sex education. Thus, when
exposed to sexually provocative situations, he might be
expected to act inappropriately. The retarded boy who has
no understanding of why he might become sexually stimulated likewise may have no understanding of why masturbation
is inappropriate. The retarded girl who has not received
skilled instructions in menstrual hygiene might not see the
importance of eliminating body odor or carefully disposing
of sanitary napkins. The school nurse with encouragement
from the health care professional can provide much of this
instruction and reinforce it on an ongoing basis. Consultation
regarding individuals as well as general information as to
instructional techniques and current teaching aids can be
offered her by the health care professional. These kinds of
services are generally received with enthusiasm and can
cement a working relationship with the school.

The mildly retarded adolescent, who frequently is more
socially acceptable and has greater access to peer contacts, is
likely to present the most concern in terms of irresponsible
sexual behavior. His need for practical information concerning reproduction and contraception presents a challenge to
professionals and parents alike. Unlike youth of average
intelligence he benefits little from nuances about appropriate
sexual behavior. Information imparted by a professional of
the same sex can be useful in that the individual can serve as
a model whose own control system can be incorporated by
the retarded youth to improve on his own lack of judgment.
School teachers and counselors are perhaps the most appropriate personnel for this role, but if professional information
and encouragement are not forthcoming they are likely to
become very frustrated.

A common request to the health care facility is for the
provision of contraception for school age retarded girls. The
concern of the school must be noted, but each decision to
employ contraceptive techniques must be individualized and

done with the cooperation of the girl and her family. The most practical method seems to be a form of the intrauterine device, but in many instances this is not deemed medically satisfactory. In some clinics oral contraceptives have been employed with reasonable success but rigid, formalized supports must be utilized concurrently. Behavior modification techniques have been found to assist the retarded girl in administering her own medication, but in some instances a parent or guardian may have to supervise the administration.

Logically, sterilization would probably be the most effective means of preventing pregnancy, but the ethical and moral consideration in terms of violating of the adolescent's rights warrant against this. In addition, there is presently a great deal of uncertainty about the legal liabilities resulting from use of sterilization procedures. Thus, although most clinics will not consider this procedure, the reasons should be explained to the parents and school officials who might be referring the child.

## The Emotionally Disturbed

School personnel on the whole do not see themselves as clinically oriented and therefore are inclined to refer the emotionally disturbed teenager for treatment at a mental health or health care facility. The school must be recognized as perhaps the most vital and strategic resource for the identification of emotionally handicapped adolescents because school personnel observe youngsters over a longer period of time and in a greater variety of situations than do persons in other professions. The emphasis placed on the patient's symptomatology at the time of his referral may or may not relate to the severity of his emotional disturbance, but respect for the school's perception of the problem is the first step toward exploring the appropriateness of the referral.

Overt patterns of truancy, suspected drug use, and

disruptive activity in the classroom are perhaps the most common types of school referrals, but withdrawal and underachievement are also noted by perceptive school personnel as reasons for referring the youth for help. Although more emphasis is usually placed by the teacher on the more disruptive patterns, and by the health personnel on patterns of withdrawal, this merely reflects the difference in role and responsibility. Health personnel usually deal with one child at a time with emphasis upon his individual health and mental health status while school personnel on the whole must focus on the adolescent's adjustment as it relates to the group. These differing viewpoints may constitute a basis for friction in the referral process, yet they can also be seen as the basis for understanding more fully the child's problems.

The breadth of professional services available in an individual health care facility will determine the extent to which it is equipped to handle the referral. Certain problems identified in school, however, will present themselves frequently in most health institutions. Three that I will discuss in more detail are: hyperactivity, school phobia, and abuse and neglect.

## HYPERACTIVITY

The hyperactive teenager is usually seen as a disruptive influence that, if not understood, will be responded to only by frustration and irritability on the teacher's part. It thus behooves the health care professional to offer sensitive guidance toward the complete evaluation of the problem and the treatment plan.

If the hyperactivity is due to neurologic impairment, the responsibility of the health care worker is first to guide the teacher toward accepting the student as an otherwise nice person who has difficulty repressing himself. Only then can the teacher begin to be receptive to offers of consultation on classroom management. School personnel in general must be treated as allied professionals who are necessary collaborators in service to neurologically impaired adolescents. Therefore, all medical information desired should be conveyed to them. My experience with the school's responses in dealing with hyperactive adolescents has demonstrated that their investment in the disabled youth seems directly proportional to my investment in explaining his condition to them.

Neurologic impairment is such a complex and frustrating condition to deal with that it may prove helpful to respond to the school with information as specific and concrete as possible. Reviewing a list of behavior patterns and subsequent diagnostic procedures can cut through some of the ambiguity. In doing so, the importance and related nature of school records, including teachers' observations, will become apparent to the conferring professional and school officials alike. Specific information and recommendations presented in accord with the philosophy of the particular health care facility can greatly facilitate communication with the school and augment their understanding of hyperactivity.

At the same time, school personnel must be helped to understand that even with the presence of neurologic factors, resulting undesirable behavior may be due to secondary emotional problems. Also important is that they note that these students are often unaware of the reasons for the negative responses they evoke in others. For these adolescents, alienation from peers can, out of frustration and discouragement, bring about resentment, hostility, and generally uncooperative behavior. The youth may well act in socially immature ways as he has not enjoyed the learning that comes from peer contact. Compensatory mechanisms for his lack of social and academic success may well present as stubbornness, lying, boasting, or withdrawal. Counseling and/or understanding responses by school and health care personnel can lessen the potential for damage threatened by emotional overlay.

For the most part special class placement is not available

to the neurologically handicapped adolescent—one of the reasons being the expectation that his hyperactivity will improve with age. This does not mean, however, that he will not continue to require close supervision, encouragement, limit-setting, and perhaps individualized scheduling. Unfortunately, so many of these youth continue to demonstrate the residual effects of a history comprised of frustrated social and educational endeavors.

Hyperactivity brought on solely by anxiety should respond to a similarly warm and limit-setting approach on the part of the teacher, but it must be understood that the youth is exhibiting this kind of behavior for the meeting of emotional needs, and that this behavior has not resulted from a neurologic problem. A psychosocial approach by qualified personnel either within the school or health care facility is indicated if this is the diagnosis. Careful evaluation need have been done previously, however, to rule out any organic factors.

Howard J. was referred to our adolescent clinic for an evaluation of what the school felt to be a strange and withdrawn behavior pattern. The family's psychosocial situation seemed noncontributory, but medical evaluation revealed some evidence of neurologic impairment. Howard had a type of neurologic deficit which resulted in poor gross motor coordination and problems in integrating detail. A referral was made to the staff psychologist who was able to delineate further the boy's behavior and learning problems. A staff conference was held subsequently during which a demonstration interview was conducted with Howard. School personnel, although invited, did not attend, but the school records were used to better understand the boy's classroom behavior. The resulting plan called for the psychologist to go to the school to assist with individualized management techniques and to offer suggestions for scheduling. It was explained that Howard had been put on medication to help him be less distractible, and his teachers were encouraged to give him direct feedback about his social behavior with peers. At last report Howard was in less trouble with other children at school. Consultation was offered on an ongoing basis.

SCHOOL PHOBIA

Although this condition is more predominant in the elementary grades, many teenagers present school phobic reactions. This reaction presents itself as an irrational aversion to school often characterized by somatic symptoms such as nausea, vomiting, headache, abdominal pain, or even low-grade fever. When this occurs at the elementary level, it is usually readily identifiable as the psychologic problem that it is; at the secondary level, however, it is often overlooked as simple truancy.

Because evaluation of physical symptomatology is the initial step to diagnosing the condition, the medical facility has a major responsibility for developing a treatment plan, and also for consulting with the school regarding dynamics and handling. As the school is the focus of the child's complaints, school personnel are often all too ready to accept responsibility—often, however, this is self-defeating. In actuality, the teenager's fear of school is a displacement of a separation fear, or an intense fear of leaving the security of home and mother—or father. The parent may seem to be cooperative in attempting to encourage attendance, but he also is reluctant about "letting go" and will likely prove himself ineffectual in facilitating the teenager's attendance.

To be therapeutic in such situations the school must be helped to clarify the areas of its own responsibility so that demands can be made of the parent. The parent must be encouraged—forcibly if necessary—to assume responsibility for the child's attendance. School personnel should be discouraged about unnecessary self-examination and the assumption of parental responsibility; this not only results in a waste of energy but can become a reason for the parent and child to avoid responsibility for their actions. The consulting medical facility can provide psychotherapy for parent and child as well as assist the school in maintaining a healthy perspective.

Susan K., age 13, was brought to our adolescent clinic for an evaluation of severe headaches that had resulted in several weeks of school absence. She presented as a childlike, withdrawn adolescent who volunteered little information. When a physical examination revealed no medical basis for the complaints, an attempt was made to understand any related psychosocial circumstances. The information revealed that the death of a grandparent had seemed to precipitate the school absences and that lingering concern about the mother's recent surgery was present also. An exceedingly dependent mother-daughter relationship was quite evident when the two were seen conjointly. Mrs. K. insisted that she was making every effort to force her daughter's attendance, yet she focused on obstacles the school was presenting that hampered her efforts. Among these were poor school bus service, racial problems in the school, and an unsympathetic school personnel. Contact with the school revealed a great deal of frustration and unnecessary self-examination on the part of school personnel.

Related school personnel were invited to a conference focused on Susan's emotional problem as well as on her general condition of school phobia. Evident was the sensitivity of the counselors but their lack of understanding in how to deal with the situation. The outcome was a plan for the school to take affirmative action with the parents, truancy action if necessary. As a concurrent measure, our clinic agreed to focus on treatment for mother and daughter to resolve the separation fears.

## NEGLECT AND ABUSE

The school plays a major role in identifying adolescents in need of protective services. Seeking help for the teenager is compatible with educational objectives since the emotional impact of serious neglect or abuse can be assumed to block or at least inhibit the adolescent's ability to perform academically.

An alert teacher, school nurse, or other school official may notice a teenager with excessive bruises or abrasions, one who sleeps in class, one who frequently is truant from school. Any or all of these may be indicators of abuse or neglect and should be evaluated further. Although incidence of actual abuse in children over age twelve is considerably reduced, related emotional, medical, and physical neglect continues and must be seen as potentially damaging as the abuse itself.

All states require that schools report suspected abuse or neglect to a local law enforcement officer, but ignorance of the law and/or fear of reprisal is great. In addition, suspected abuse also has a strong emotional impact upon all those who must deal with it; negative or punitive feelings toward the suspected abuser are common and should be recognized. Denial of these feelings may result in denial of the possibility of abuse and thus the exploration and reporting of it; school personnel should be helped to understand this underlying psychologic possibility. The health care facility thus can play a major role in terms of educating and reassuring school personnel who are in a position to report abuse or neglect situations. More commonly, however, the health care professional collaborates with the school in initiation of protective action. Many school officials may be hesitant to identify what they feel may be abuse or neglect, but confirmation by the hospital or clinic encourages them to do so. The reverse can be true as well; the school can often clarify the circumstances surrounding a probable neglect or abuse situation that might come to the attention of the health care worker.

Incest and sexual abuse of adolescents are much more common occurrences than often realized. Dr. Vincent DeFrancis, director of the Children's Division of the American Human Association, has estimated that about 100,000 children throughout the country are subjected to sexual abuse each year.[6] The symptoms that are observable in school are more complex than those of physical abuse, because guilt and anxiety over the experience can be expressed in any number of ways. It is important for school personnel to recognize the incidence of sexual abuse, and to be alert and sensitive to the possibilities of its existence in the student population.

Although the preceding information seems to exclude the teenager as informant, this is not meant to be the case. I should point out, however, that in any experience with abused and neglected teenagers the tendency on their part to conceal information is great. In some cases this is related to a fear of actual physical reprisal but in more instances to a seldom acknowledged, but greater feared, loss of love. This is illustrated by the following:

> Amy P., age 13, was brought to the Emergency Room by the school nurse. She had come to school with a severe cut and bruises about her leg which she stated had been caused by a two-year-old cousin having hit her with a belt. The nurse was concerned that the family had not provided medical treatment for the cut, and when she could not reach them by telephone, decided to initiate the request for treatment herself. Other factors had influenced her decision to bring Amy to the Emergency Room as well. Apparently, Amy had continued to present in school with numerous scratches or abrasions on her body, and had repeatedly fallen asleep in class. The nurse, in addition, had had difficulty in determining the relationships of the people whom Amy called her family.

> When I spoke with her Amy exhibited extreme withdrawal and anxiety. Only after a great deal of support and repeated statements that I didn't think a two-year-old could hurt her leg that way did Amy tell me her uncle had hit her with a belt. Apparently severe beatings had gone on for some time, and she was extremely unhappy with her living situation. She had rather clearly been fearful of exposing the uncle's maltreatment for fear of reprisal.

> When her aunt and uncle with whom Amy was living were contacted, it was learned that Amy had been left with them a year and a half previously by her mother, a traveling minister. Although the aunt denied that Amy had in any way been maltreated, she was extremely hostile and described her niece as a burden to her and her husband. Amy was not sent home from the Emergency Room that day; an emergency court order was obtained and Amy was placed in a protective foster home.

This chapter discussed the more common physical and emotional problems of adolescents and the respective roles of the school and the health care facility in recognizing and managing them. The interrelationship of both facilities is stressed in terms of its importance in providing more fully for the health care needs of the teenager.

REFERENCES

1.  Harris H: The range of psychosomatic disorders in adolescents. In Howells JG (ed): Modern Perspectives in Adolescent Psychiatry. New York, Brunner/Mazel, 1971, p 239
2.  Swift CR: Report on a Pilot Study. Juvenile Diabetes: Adjustment and Emotional Problems, Proceedings of a Workshop Sponsored by the US Public Health Service, et al, Held at Princeton, NJ, April 22–23, 1963, p 23
3.  Duckett C: Fighting sickle cell disease. Children, Vol 18, No. 6, Nov–Dec 1971, p 230
4.  Hathaway W: Education and Health of the Partially Seeing Child. New York, Columbia U Press, 1954, p 41
5.  Hammar SL, Barnard KE: The mentally retarded adolescent: a review of the characteristics and problems of 44 non-institutionalized adolescent retardates. Pediatrics, Vol 38, No. 5, Nov 1966, p 850
6.  Fontana VJ: Somewhere a Child Is Crying. New York, Macmillan, 1973, p 96

BIBLIOGRAPHY

Auslander G: A conceptual framework for the use of consultation in the schools. Unpublished Paper, The Jane Addams School of Social Work, University of Illinois at Chicago, 1969
Duckett CL: Caring for children with sickle cell anemia. Children Vol 18, No. 6(November–December, 1971)
Fontana VJ: Somewhere a Child Is Crying. New York, Macmillan, 1973
Hammar SL, Barnard KE: The mentally retarded adolescent: a review of the characteristics and problems of 44 non-institutionalized adolescent retardates. Pediatrics, Vol 38, Nov 1966, pp 845–856
Hathaway W: Education and Health of the Partially Seeing Child, 3rd ed. New York, Columbia U Press, 1954
Howells JG (ed): Modern Perspectives in Adolescent Psychiatry. New York, Brunner/Mazel, 1971
Kaplan L: Education and Mental Health. New York, Harper & Row, 1971
Nemir A: The School Health Program. Philadelphia, Saunders, 1965
Shirley HF: Pediatric Psychiatry. Cambridge, Harvard U Press, 1963

Swift CR: Report on a Pilot Study. Juvenile Diabetes: Adjustment and
Emotional Problems, Proceedings of a Workshop Sponsored by the
United States Public Health Service, et al, held at Princeton, NJ,
April 22–23, 1963

# 5

# Obesity in Teenage Girls

JANET FENDER

## AN APPROACH TO THE OBESE TEENAGE GIRL

Although estimates vary as to the number of female adolescents who are considered obese, it is well known that adolescent obesity is a prevalent condition that is potentially damaging to the young girl's psychosocial development,[1] and is essentially untreatable if she remains obese past the adolescent period.[2]

It is therefore imperative that research be directed toward improving treatment methods for the problem of adolescent female obesity, for "the present treatment methods have been disappointing in their effectiveness for all age groups, but especially for the adolescent."[3]

For the above general reasons and for the specific reason that we* were confronted with a group of unhappy, obese

*"We" refers to Audrey Kalafatich, R.N., M.S., with whom I participated in this approach, and myself.

adolescent girls who were not responding to a conventional weight reduction regime consisting of a low calorie diet, increased physical activity, and anorexigenic agents, we felt that it was essential to develop a new approach to this problem. In the following pages I shall describe our approach used with a small group of obese female adolescents in an outpatient setting. First some background information is necessary in order to clarify the basic reasons for the failure of traditional treatment approaches as applied to the adolescent, and also to provide a rationale for our particular approach.

## Background Literature

In surveying the literature I found mention of numerous, complexly interrelated factors that predispose to, precipitate, and perpetuate obesity. However, it is neither relevant to our study nor within the scope of this paper to describe all of these. It is essential, however, to have a general appreciation of the complexity of variables involved in order to understand why the results of traditional treatment approaches are often dismal, especially for the adolescent.

Traditional approaches for treating obesity, decreased caloric intake and/or increased caloric output, are based on the statement that the primary cause of obesity is caloric intake in excess of caloric output: thus, " . . . the excess calories are stored as fat."[4] Although this long-established concept is true, it often oversimplifies the problem, and leads to oversimplified approaches to it which ultimately leads to failure.

The following discusses the basis for these traditional treatment approaches and their success rate as applied to the adolescent on an outpatient basis.

## DECREASED CALORIC INTAKE

Most of the attention in treatment of obesity has been directed toward and concerned with dietary intake. This thinking has led to the use of a variety of dietary regimes and anorexigenic agents. These treatment approaches are based on the premise that the primary etiologic and perpetuating factor of adolescent obesity is overeating. However, it has been stated in the literature that, for the most part, obesity in adolescents is not caused by excessive eating. In fact, it has been shown that the average daily caloric intake of the obese adolescent is the same or lower than that of her nonobese peers.[3(p 3)] These are significant facts that cast some doubt on the value of decreasing the adolescent's caloric intake as a means of correcting her problem.

The dietary approach has often failed because it is not directed at the factor (decreased energy output) responsible for the causation and maintenance of obesity in most adolescents, and also because of the adolescent's inability to maintain the diet on an outpatient basis. Some of the probable reasons for this lack of follow-through are as follows:

1. The medically supervised diet, because of the basic concern for meeting the nutritional needs of the growing adolescent, is often extremely slow in providing results. Adolescents are by nature very present-oriented and thus want and expect quick results. They easily become discouraged with a diet and give up. Thus, the adolescent needs to establish a therapeutic relationship with a health worker in order to have a source of continuous, understanding support and encouragement which is crucial in sustaining her interest and motivation. On an outpatient basis, however, with the typical infrequency of visits and the lack of continuity with one person, this source is often lacking.

2. A diet is generally very negative in its orientation. It stresses what *not* to eat. Adolescents generally find this negative advice very difficult to follow because it often fails to incorporate enough allowances for the typical food fads of this age group. Adolescence is a time when it is very important to be liked and accepted by one's peers, and diet restrictions further exclude the obese adolescent from her nonobese peers, thus emphasizing her differences. This negative advice is also difficult for her to follow because it deprives her of even the normal quota of oral and social satisfaction provided by food without substituting other gratifications in its place.

There are many methods of reducing dietary intake other than the most common—the low calorie medically supervised diet used principally in our outpatient clinic. However, the others have many of the same drawbacks as those mentioned above, plus that of not adequately meeting the nutritional and energy needs of the growing adolescent.

I do not want to be completely negative about the value of some type of diet therapy in the treatment program for the obese adolescent. The disadvantages I have described apply when a diet is used as the sole treatment approach on an outpatient basis. However, there have been cited in the literature some successes, especially when the dietary regime is (1) only part of the total treatment regime, (2) used in some sort of an inpatient setting, and (3) when the emphasis is on the positive, normal aspects of the diet such as is used at Camp Seascape.[5] Even so, treatment by dietary management has yielded poor long-term results in most cases.[3 (pp 14, 15)]

Also aimed primarily at decreasing intake are anorexigenic agents. Aside from the fact they are not directed at the factor responsible for and perpetuating adolescent obesity, use of these agents has other disadvantages. The literature supports the fact that, if used, they should be only a minor adjunct in the total treatment regime. Also, the adolescent should be carefully screened before being placed on them and followed closely with medical supervision. Some of the disadvantages are: (1) they can be habituating, (2) they have many adverse side effects, (3) they lose their effectiveness after long-term use, and (4) they are often viewed by the adolescent as magical, melting away pounds with little effort.[6] The adolescent often has unrealistic expectations concerning the benefits of these agents, thus creating a situation where sole responsibility of weight loss is placed on an external source. The individual's internal motivation, which is one of the essential ingredients for successful weight loss, is thereby mitigated.

## INCREASED CALORIC OUTPUT

As previously stated, the only way to lose weight is to decrease caloric intake and/or to increase caloric output. Let us now turn our attention to the treatment method of increasing energy expenditure through increasing one's level of physical activity.

One of the most neglected factors in the incidence of obesity is inactivity rather than hyperphagia. It has been shown that the obese female adolescent spends a significantly lesser amount of time than her respective nonobese controls in activities involving any amount of energy expenditure.[7]

These studies have suggested that inactivity might be an important factor in the development and perpetuation of the obese state. In other words, physical inactivity rather than overeating appears to be responsible for the positive energy balance.

A factor which has possibly resulted in the neglect of exercise as an influence in weight control is the common misconception that with all increased energy expenditure there is a corresponding increase in intake. This is not true. Moderate exercise does not increase the appetite. It has also been demonstrated that those who exercise within a normal range of activity eat somewhat less than those who do not exercise at all.[4](p 141)

Another common fallacy advanced to justify neglecting exercise is that physical activity consumes very little energy. This is inaccurate; it has been shown that significant calorie amounts can be expended during moderate exercise sessions with no comparable increase in caloric intake.[8]

It seems, therefore, that if we treated adolescent obesity by increasing their physical activity level they would achieve weight loss. Although this is essentially true, the success rate of this method on an outpatient basis has been very disappointing.[3](pp 33, 34, 35) WHY?(1) Again, treatment on an out patient basis simply does not provide the adolescent with enough sustaining encouragement and support; (2) although the adolescent is given a prescription of increased activity, the implementation and follow-through of the exercise program is the sole responsibility of the individual. This requires a major change in the adolescent's daily habits and these changes are difficult to achieve and maintain because of the lack of gratification inherent in the exercises themselves; (3) weight loss with this method is slow. I have already mentioned that adolescents tend to desire quick results or they become discouraged. Thus, any stimulus for follow-through is lacking.

In short, increased physical activity can undoubtedly be beneficial on an outpatient basis, but too much is left to chance, and the factors that contribute to the obese adolescent's inactivity are ignored.

THE MISSING LINK

It is evident that to treat the problem of adolescent obesity successfully, it is *not* sufficient just to know that the primary contributing and perpetuating factor is inactivity, and that treatment should be aimed at increasing energy expenditure.

If the solution were as simple as that, we would not have the failure rate that we have. Also essential is that we understand the adolescent who is obese, the psychosocial effects of obesity on her, and how these tend to perpetuate the condition and thus contribute to the difficulty of alleviating it.

To understand the delicate interplay of simultaneously being an adolescent and being obese, I found it necessary to explore the typical developmental tasks and psychosocial characteristics and needs of this particular age group.

The central task of adolescence is to develop an identity. Adolescence is a time of increased awareness of and concern about one's body. The attitudes which the adolescent develops about her own physical appearance are to a great extent derived from her comparisons with and feedback from other people. The "other people" include our entire culture, since the adolescent's concept of herself is largely determined by what is acceptable therein.[9] Our culture has generally a derogatory and unaccepting attitude toward obesity and thus toward those who are obese. The obese adolescent sees reminders of this everywhere. Television, the press, the fashion industry all overemphasize the desirability of a trim figure. Unfortunately, the image that the adolescent derives of herself physically is an important factor in the development of her self-image or identity.[10]

But even more important in the development of the adolescent's self-image is the reaction of her peers to her appearance. Peers are an extremely important influence in the adolescent's life. To a significant degree, physical appearance is an important factor in how the individual is evaluated by her peers. To be different from one's peers is often to be inferior and to be rejected.

Thus the negative attitude with which significant others view her physical appearance affects adversely the way in which the obese adolescent views herself. This generally unfavorable and unaccepting atmosphere in which the adolescent has to live has many negative social and psychologic effects on her.

## SOCIAL EFFECTS

The obese adolescent is often socially disapproved of, ridiculed, and rejected by her peers. Yet many of the adolescent's developmental tasks and needs must be worked through and resolved with the support of peer group association. The obese adolescent is to a great extent denied these healthy, normal, social learning opportunities. Thus, she is blocked or handicapped in her attempt to establish a well-adjusted identity, to successfully achieve her developmental tasks, and to meet her basic human needs of approval, acceptance, love, and so forth.

"Every adolescent has a need for a sense of her own worth and anything that tends to make her feel inadequate or inferior is apt to be met promptly with some kind of defensive reaction."[11] The obese adolescent frequently reacts by isolating herself and withdrawing from the unfavorable social atmosphere.

## PSYCHOLOGIC EFFECTS

As stated previously, the obese teenager's self-image is largely an internalization of the social attitudes toward her obesity. It is therefore not surprising that the obese adolescent often has a negative self-image. This is confirmed by psychologic tests which show that she often has feelings of low self-esteem, inadequacy, inferiority, low self-acceptance, and low self-confidence.[12]

Thus, in conclusion, the negative social attitudes toward obesity lead to the development of adverse psychosocial consequences for the obese adolescent, which lead to withdrawal and isolation. The effect is a decreased activity level which perpetuates the obese condition, and ultimately results in the establishment of a vicious cycle.

In summary, overeating is usually not the primary contributing factor in the development of obesity in the adolescent. To focus treatment primarily on decreasing caloric intake would necessitate a very severe restriction of calories. Only this way can a daily caloric intake be achieved that is less than the daily low energy output of the typical obese teenager. But this type of treatment regime would not only adversely affect the adolescent's growth, it would be almost impossible for her to maintain.

### Our Approach

From reviewing the literature and from experience, a program for obese teenage girls based on dietary restriction did not seem feasible. Langdell[13] offered a diagram of the circular nature of the problem (Fig. 1). He also proposed that if the system were to be broken in two places, the cycle would be stopped.

We decided to try to break the cycle in the area of underactivity by providing a treatment regime that included

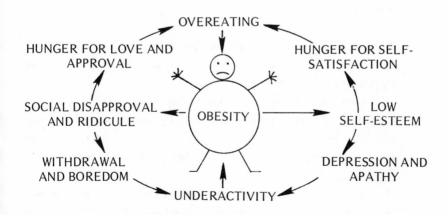

FIG. 1. The vicious cycle in female adolescent obesity. (From Langdell: In Szurek (ed): Psychosomatic Disorders and Mental Retardation, 1968. Courtesy of Science and Behavior Books.)

increased activity and by increasing each girl's self-esteem. Because of the psychosocial factors that seem to perpetuate the inactivity pattern, we decided that a simple prescription of increased activity was not the sole answer. We therefore attempted to provide an accepting, nonthreatening atmosphere in which to support and to encourage the adolescent in her development of a more satisfying and realistic self-image, and in her development of a more normal, healthy pattern of social adaptation. At the same time, a regular program of group activity in a social setting was used as a means to help the adolescent gain confidence and enjoyment in active physical participation, and as a means to increase her energy expenditure.

Our main emphasis was not on weight loss because of the short duration of our program but rather on providing the adolescent with the means necessary for *eventual* weight reduction. Others have supported our general contention that an improvement in body image and thus self-esteem is important in regard to the initiation of more satisfying psychosocial adaptations which should ultimately result in weight reduction.[14]

OBJECTIVES

At this point it is necessary to describe the framework upon which we structured our particular approach so that we may clarify our objectives.

Our objectives were based upon the framework of providing an atmosphere in which to aid in modifying the negative psychosocial and inactivity factors that tend to perpetuate the vicious cycle of obesity. Our objectives were to provide:

1. An experience of group social interaction and discussion in order to (a) provide an opportunity to share common problems and thus to derive mutual help and support in dealing with them; (b) to gain beginning self-awareness,

self-understanding, and self-acceptance; and (c) to gain confidence in social and interpersonal situations.

2. Constructive experiences which would assist these girls in recognition, acceptance, and mobilization of their positive assets in order to improve their self-image.

3. Opportunities for participation in a variety of group and individual physical activities in an effort to (a) enhance the girl's enjoyment of and confidence in different active pursuits; (b) to help the girls become aware of the important use of activity in the energy balance; and (c) to encourage them to continue this pattern of increased activity in their everyday lives.

## METHODS

The general methods that were used in carrying out our particular objectives are as follows:

1. Group discussion
2. Group activity
3. Individual consultation

## Sample Population

Now I would like to delve further into the specifics of our particular approach by describing first the composition of our group.

Initially, letters of invitation, which generally explained the proposed group, were sent out to most of the girls who were presently coming to the outpatient adolescent clinic for their weight problem. The only girls not invited were those whose obesity was caused primarily by either physiologic or psychologic factors. We chose to eliminate these two factors from our sample group in order to have some control over the many possible contributing variables and also because these two factors in particular must be dealt with prior to active individual participation. For example, when emotional problems are the major cause of the obesity, concurrent overeating often aids the individual in meeting her basic needs and helps her to maintain an emotional balance. Any attempts to remove this basic source of satisfaction without concurrent intensive psychotherapeutic support often throw this particular individual into severe mental disequilibrium.[15] On the other hand, when organic problems are the cause of the obesity, it is quite easy for the person to deny any individual responsibility for her state and thus the internal motivation necessary for sustained interest in a program is lacking. Until the physiologic causes are controlled and the individual sincerely accepts that her obesity is now *her* problem to deal with, it is futile to expect follow-through in any treatment program.

Some other characteristics of our sample group are as follows. Inclusion in the group was not dependent on any specific degree of obesity, even though there are a variety of standards of measurement that can be utilized. Essentially, the girls defined themselves as overweight, and all were significantly overweight by observation. They were between eleven and seventeen years of age, although the majority were over fourteen. All were from lower socioeconomic backgrounds but from different races.

Fifteen of the forty girls originally contacted expressed an interest in the group and were subsequently given specific details as to the time and location of the first meeting.

We felt very strongly that participation in this program should be strictly voluntary and thus no pressure for involvement was applied. One of the typical struggles of adolescence is with the need to be independent and often, if *forced* to comply, they will not cooperate. Also, those who volunteer are known to be more apt to profit from the experience. The individual who recognizes her need for help seems to accept greater responsibility for improvement.[16] As mentioned previously, internal motivation for weight loss is an essential ingredient for success.

### Group Approach

I will now describe the specific methods by which we carried out our general objectives by explaining first the reasons for a group approach and then by describing our initial and subsequent sessions.

We felt that a group approach was particularly appropriate because peers are typically the adolescent's primary source of communication and support. Other studies which have described the highest degree of success (both in weight management and in improved psychosocial adjustment) have been group efforts where others were present with similar problems.[14(p 33)]

During the adolescent period, when peer acceptance and approval are very important, it is very supportive to discover that fellow peers have the same kinds of problems. Discovering the problems she has in common with others helps each adolescent to feel that she belongs and that she is more readily understood. This discovery also helps to create a safe, accepting atmosphere in which it is easier to be open and honest in sharing feelings without fear of ridicule or being different.

This feeling of alliance with a peer group is especially important for the obese adolescent who often has experienced only rejection by such significant others.

### INITIAL MEETING

The first meeting of a group is very important in terms of setting the tone for subsequent sessions. Several factors influence this and location is one of these. The location of our initial meeting was in a building next to the outpatient clinic so that the site would be easily accessible and familiar to all the girls. We wanted to decrease anxiety as much as possible by reducing the number of unknowns that are inherent in any new situation. However, we did not want to meet in the teenage clinic itself because we did not want the girls to start out with any preconceived notions. In other words, we did not want the girls to transfer possible negative attitudes about their past experiences with weight loss to this new opportunity.

Another influencing factor in setting tone is the nature of the meeting place. We wanted the atmosphere of this first meeting to be informal, warm, and private. Thus we chose a small, quiet room and arranged the chairs in a circle, in order to enhance visual and verbal interaction.

Most of the girls were unfamiliar with this type of group experience and so we expected that feelings of anxiety would be high. Our expectation was realized, for in the beginning the girls were very hesitant to verbalize and demonstrated many nervous gestures. To initiate some interaction, we began by introducing ourselves and by giving a short autobiography. It was important to establish at the outset that we expected and wanted mutual sharing of ideas, feelings, and so forth. We encouraged the girls to follow our example and soon many barriers were down because the girls realized that they attended the same schools, had similiar interests, and such.

At the first meeting it is also beneficial to clarify objectives and the means of achieving these so as to provide a common workable framework and to decrease individual anxiety. In discussing the goals, however, we were very careful to keep them fairly general to give the girls the impression that our program was flexible and that they themselves would ultimately be deciding on the specifics as their needs came to light. From the very beginning we wanted the girls to feel like active participants in the decision making process. This we felt would enhance their feeling that the group was theirs and would increase their inner sense of commitment and responsibility.

Basically, we stated that the group's purpose was for sharing the common problems and concerns of being overweight, the goal being that of arriving at some workable solutions to these problems through the avenues of group discussion and group participation in activities. At no time did we mention any specific achievements, especially that of weight loss, to be one of the prime objectives, for we did not want the girls to feel any specific external pressure for achievement, or to measure the worth of the group in terms of this standard. Such not only would tend to result in a feeling of failure if not achieved but also would tend to make the motivating factor an external one—that of pleasing *us*. Instead, we hoped that each girl could, at her own pace and in her own way, gain some positive psychosocial benefits from this experience.

Also, by being flexible we hoped to avoid the authoritarian struggle. Especially, when working with adolescents with their vacillating dependency-independency needs, it is difficult but very essential to arrive at the right balance of structure. "Effective structuring contributes to the therapeutic climate; overstructuring and rigid rules interfere with it."[16](p 113)

Next, we encouraged the girls to ask any clarifying questions. These stimulated discussion about the length and frequency of meetings. As a group we compromised and came to an agreement to meet every Tuesday from 3 p.m. to 5 p.m. for eight weeks. The length and frequency of sessions should be adapted to the group's overall maturity and needs, and also should be appropriate for meeting the stated objectives.[17]

At this point we felt the need to emphasize a few basic technical rules so that the group could function as smoothly and productively as possible. We told the girls that we would like to see them continue with the group if they so decided but that we expected them to be on time and to attend every session. It has been documented that those who attend regularly tend to profit most from the experience. [16](p 102) We also stated that no new members could be added in subsequent weeks. Because our group was of short duration, we felt that the addition of new members would be disruptive to the ongoing therapeutic progress of those initially present.

Up to this point *we* had been doing most of the talking so as to decrease anxiety and to clarify the situation. By now the girls seemed more comfortable and so were encouraged to discuss their feelings and concerns about their weight. From here on we became more active *listeners* than authoritarian participants. Typically, the adolescent is extremely preoccupied with self. Because of this trait, no female in any other age group is as likely to quickly form a close and therapeutically useful relationship with the adult whom she feels is genuinely concerned about her, and who unconditionally respects her as a person of worth. This requires an active, interested, nonjudgmental listener.

Our purpose was not to give all-knowing advice but rather to support and encourage the girls in the identification and the verbalization of their feelings and concerns. This we hoped would aid them in moving through the problem solving process, and in the direction of developing healthier behavior and attitudes toward themselves and their obesity problems.

Adolescents are the best sources of information about themselves. Through informal discussion and observation of their behavior, we had the opportunity to learn firsthand about these girls' feelings, concerns, and interests rather than to proceed on our own preconceived notions. The girls generally voiced many of the concerns that were identified previously in this chapter in conjunction with obesity in adolescence. The youngsters were negative in most facets of their self-appraisal, voiced concern over their lack of boyfriends, seemed to expect and feel they deserved social ridicule and disapproval, and had few activities outside the home. They were generally dissatisfied with themselves and wanted to change their appearance. However, many of the girls expressed unrealistic expectations and ambitions concerning weight loss. For example, several wanted to lose weight so that they could become models and actresses. Therefore, throughout the course of the sessions we worked with the girls on developing short-term, realistic goals. We felt that successful achievement of attainable goals would sustain their motivation over a long period of time.

## SUBSEQUENT SESSIONS

After the second session the group had stabilized at six participants. These girls continued to attend regularly until termination. Six to eight members are generally cited as an appropriate size for an adolescent group.

An effort was made to contact by telephone the other initial attenders in order to demonstrate our continued interest and support. Our goal was not to coerce these girls into attending but rather to intervene if extraneous problems such as transportation or misconceptions regarding the group were the obstacles. Also, we wanted to let them know that we respected whatever decisions they made and that future opportunities would be open to them whenever they deemed them appropriate. We certainly did not want to add to the feelings of rejection that many of these girls realistically experience from external sources.

During the following seven sessions, a variety of activities and discussions were pursued; these will be described more specifically in the following sections.

*Activity Sessions.*   The activities engaged in had to be acceptable to the group members if they were going to benefit from them, so it was always a group decision as to what we would do. These plans were made the previous week so that the girls could be prepared, and so that the activity would reflect their current needs and interests. During our subsequent sessions we engaged in such activities as swimming, volleyball, basketball, and bike riding.

Many of the girls, because of feelings of self-consciousness and fear of social ridicule and failure, had withdrawn from physical activity situations. By recognition of the factors involved in the individual's lack of follow-through with the previously discussed outpatient activity program, we realized that a structured environment was necessary, at least initially, in order to encourage each girl's participation in a physical activity program. Our structured group activity program provided them with a relatively nonthreatening and supportive opportunity in which to experiment safely.

With safe opportunities to discover her capabilities the adolescent is able to gain in her understanding of herself and increase her self-confidence. Thus, we hoped that the girls would come to recognize their abilities, would be able to derive a sense of gratification and enjoyment from activities, and that ultimately these realizations might overcome their withdrawal from active participation.

The group's support seemed to overcome initial shyness. We were active participants in all the activities and thus were able to intervene therapeutically on an individual basis whenever the need arose. For example, one of the girls expressed a desire to learn how to dive, but her perception of how she would look as expressed in her statement, "I'll just look like some baby whale when I make my big splash," thwarted her initial attempt. I also enjoy diving, and so with my support and encouragement the girl finally made the attempt, and during the rest of that session we practiced our diving together. I believe that once this youngster realized what an enjoyable and safe experience diving was, her initial apprehension was lessened to where she could follow through with her expressed desire.

The girls were often very self-belittling and either would not or could not recognize their realistic aptitudes and abilities in physical skills. To help them to recognize and to accept their positive assets we repeatedly acknowledged,

praised, encouraged, and reinforced these. "To build confidence, to strengthen their egos, they need . . . the happy
experience and the recognition which achievement and
success can bring."[4 (p 16)] All of us benefit from praise and
success, but these are especially important to the obese
adolescent, who often receives criticism and experiences
failure.

To aid with this positive self-realization we encouraged
the more skilled of the girls to help the less skilled. Helping
others enhances one's own self-respect because one can feel
genuinely needed and appreciated. This is especially important for the adolescent who relies so heavily on peers for
prestige and recognition. For example, one girl who showed
ability in serving the ball during a volleyball game was
encouraged to share her talent by assisting the other girls to
improve this particular skill. Thus each girl was helped to
realize that in some areas she had more to offer others but in
other areas she had more to receive from others. Hopefully,
this aided the girls toward developing a realistic self-appraisal
not only of their talents but also of their deficits.

However, all of the girls' attempts were worthy of
recognition. We wished to reinforce the idea that to make the
effort was what was important; that achievement need not be
outstanding in order to be recognized, nor that anyone had
to be extremely talented in an activity to gain satisfaction,
recognition, and enjoyment from it.

All of the activity sessions were set in a variety of
real-life situations. We felt that being in real-life situations
from the start would aid the girls in continuing to pursue the
activities in their daily lives after the group's termination.
Hence continuity of increased physical activity participation
in daily life was also explicitly discussed. For example, the
girl who enjoyed diving was encouraged to pursue the activity
at her local pool. Another girl who enjoyed our basketball
sessions was encouraged to try out for her school's intramural
team. We also encouraged all the girls to participate in their

physical education classes, which many of them admittedly were not doing. Hopefully, our activity program was helping the girls to gain confidence in and desire for increased physical participation with their nonobese peers, and with less sensitivity about their obesity and skill deficiencies. Ultimately, we hoped to extend the benefits of this group beyond its termination.

We also stressed, especially by example, the little day-by-day ways to increase one's activity. For example, we always used steps instead of elevators, and we would walk rather than ride in cars whenever feasible. Many of the girls did not realize that weight increases result not only from overeating but also from underactivity. We tried to emphasize the value of physical activity in a weight reduction program which also helped the girls to realize that increased physical activity often made weight reduction easier as well as more fun.

These activity sessions often stimulated topics for discussion. The diving episode allowed the girl to ventilate her feelings about her self-perceptions and also led to a discussion about what type of bathing suit would be most flattering to her figure and where she might obtain one inexpensively. Relating to each other in real-life situations seemed to help the girls' feelings, needs, and interests to surface. We found that they had much more difficulty discussing their feelings when we set aside a session for general discussion without having any concrete discussion topic or situation to which to respond. So we tried to allow time for discussion after or during each activity session so that feelings and thoughts could flow more easily since they were current and the need was greatest at this point.

"Talking is usually good for intellectual understanding of personal experience, but it often is not as effective for helping a person to experience—to feel. Combining the non-verbal with the verbal seems to create a much more powerful tool for cultivating human growth."[18] Thus the combination of activity and discussion was a very beneficial experience for our group because it seemed to aid the girls in recognizing and identifying their feelings, something which is necessary before they can be dealt with constructively.

*Body-Image Improvement Sessions.* These sessions included discussions and demonstrations on grooming which included hair styles, makeup, and fashion. Again the girls decided on the topics so that the sessions would be more relevant to their current needs.

Adolescents have increased awareness of and concern about their physical appearance. Throughout our interaction with the girls during the eight weeks we frequently heard them remark about their various appearance deficits but seldom about their assets. Thus we hoped that these sessions would aid the girls to recognize and accept their positive assets and how they could utilize these to improve their appearance. Our aim was to help the girls find ways in which they could feel good about their bodies now and thereby improve their self-image.

For these sessions the girls brought in wigs, makeup, and pictures of clothing that they felt would be flattering to their figures. Then they experimented with different hair styles and makeup and would get appropriate feedback from the others as to what was most flattering. In a noncritical and supportive way we discussed which features were assets and should be highlighted and which should be toned down. This aided the girls in gaining a total, realistic impression of their physical appearance.

Another study had shown that much attention should be paid to the issue of body-image and self-image improvement. The hypothesis was that successful weight losers had improved their body-image which in turn improved their self-image, and this in turn helped them to keep their weight down. This study, therefore, highly encouraged a body-image improvement program which would include sessions on grooming, fashion, and so forth.[14(p 35)]

That this approach is helpful was indicated also in our study. Several of the girls consistently paid more attention to their outer appearance and incorporated many of the group's improvement suggestions after such sessions. We felt this to be an important indication of each girl's increased positive self-esteem and thus we reinforced such positive behavior toward the self.

*Diet.* In our particular approach, minimal emphasis was given to diet instruction, since most recent studies show that adolescents usually do not have hyperphagia associated with their obesity. Also, since all the girls in our group were continuing to see their dietician, we felt that she had more expert knowledge in this area and we did not want to duplicate efforts unnecessarily. However, since we did realize that adequate nutritional education was one of the factors essential to a well-balanced weight reduction program, we encouraged the girls to continue to see their dietician and we relayed to her potential problem areas as they were identified. To emphasize to the girls the value of such professional help, we invited the clinic dietician to be our consultant, and she attended several of our sessions.

We intervened in this area in very simple, practical ways as the need arose. For example, after several of our physical activity sessions the entire group would meet for refreshments consisting of diet soft drinks. We also found that many of the girls had a poor concept of what were high-caloric foods. We therefore generally discussed types of foods high in calories and identified specific low-caloric snack foods. However, we did not want to relay the impression that the typical food crazes of adolescence were "forbidden fruit" because it is well known that many adolescent social sessions involve eating such foods. To help these girls realize that they need not totally abstain (which would be unrealistic to expect) and that they need not withdraw from such social gatherings, we stressed that some of all foods may be eaten, but in varying amounts, depending upon the type of food.

We were able to demonstrate that one could participate in a social gathering without totally ignoring diet restrictions when we celebrated a group member's birthday. Our refreshments for the occasion were generally low in calories, but high-caloric foods were available for the girls to sample in moderate amounts.

*Weighing-In.*    Although originally we did not plan to incorporate regular recording of weight as part of our program, many of the girls insisted that they be weighed. Thus the girls were weighed when and if they so desired. Very little significance was attached to this procedure because of the possible negative consequences previously discussed. The session was private and no one's weight gains or losses were discussed publicly. When the girls lost some weight or stayed the same from one week to the next, we discussed possible reasons for this success in order to reinforce individual efforts. Any weight gains were discussed by citing possible reasons and positive, practical ways to control them. We thereby hoped to reinforce the fact that the girls were unconditionally accepted by us as individuals regardless of their weight, and to reinforce feelings of self-worth.

The weigh-in procedure also gave us the opportunity to discuss realistic expectations for weight reduction. A loss of no more than two pounds per week was considered realistic. Again we emphasized that no approach to weight control would "magically" cause pounds to melt away but that, instead, regular weight loss would require a great deal of consistent work and effort. We emphasized this repeatedly because the typical adolescent often has unrealistic expectations for quick results and thus easily tends to become discouraged and give up.

*Termination.*    The aspect of the group's termination was dealt with from the start. Advance preparation and planning for termination is especially important for the adolescent because her dependency needs are often transferred to and satisfied by a significant external source, such as a peer group. They must be gradually weaned from these attachments because at this age they are particularly vulnerable to feelings of rejection and desertion that would be brought on by abrupt termination. From the very beginning, therefore, the specific duration of the group was discussed and periodically, the number of sessions remaining was mentioned.

In addition, to aid the girls in dealing with their feelings about termination, our last group session was devoted to a discussion of this. At that time the girls asked about a possible future obesity group. From this we gathered that some of them desired some future follow-up. Although we were unable to make any definite commitments about future groups, the opportunity for the girls to consult with us individually at the clinic was offered. Thus, some provision for long-term supportive maintenance was made available, but only if the individual felt the need for such services and took the initiative to obtain them.

We also provided for smooth continuity and consistent future follow-up by consulting with our co-workers during the planning and implementation stages of our group, and by keeping them informed of each girl's individual progress. Thus others in the clinic would be generally familiar with the problems in the event that neither of us were available in the future.

All of the members of our group were concurrently seeing their physician, social worker, and/or dietician in regard to their weight problem. Our goal all along was not to reject or undermine these present therapeutic regimes but rather to supplement them. At termination we held a panel discussion in which we described our particular approach to all our co-workers from the teenage clinic. Two of the girls from our group also participated in this discussion. Finally, a written summary of each girl's progress during the course of our sessions was added to her clinic charts.

As previously discussed, self-image improvement is necessary for successful weight loss. Our approach was therefore aimed at modifying the negative psychosocial perpetuating factors of obesity. We wished to aid the girls in developing more healthy, adaptive attitudes and behaviors so that they could independently gain satisfaction in meeting their typical, basic psychosocial needs. Our goal was to help them feel good about themselves right now so that the sustaining motivation necessary for eventual successful weight loss would be internal. We attempted to accomplish these results by providing opportunities in which the girls could increase their self-confidence and pleasure in physical activity; improve their skills in social and interpersonal relationships through peer group involvement; and improve their body-image

Although we did not use specific, objective tools to measure improvement in these areas, we did get general, subjective indications of such improvement. Several of the older teenagers seemed to gain the most in terms of visible, demonstrable improvement. These girls were consistently more aware of their appearance, did manage to lose some weight, seemed to incorporate more physical activity into their daily lives, and also were active participants in the group discussions and activities. Although the younger members did not demonstrate such visible evidence of progress, they attended consistently, participated actively, and seemed to enjoy themselves. Perhaps they were not quite ready or mature enough to benefit fully, but at least the sessions may have provided them with some immediate positive benefits, such as association with peers. Hopefully, from participation in *our* program they might later avail themselves of a similar opportunity when their motivation and needs are greater.

Thus, for the purpose of our group, weight loss was not a good criterion by which to judge success, although it is the most objective and commonly used evidence of such.

## Limitations

From our initial attempt to provide a workable approach to the obesity problems of adolescent girls we concluded that some modifications of our original plan would be necessary in future endeavors. For example, we would plan our approach in terms of a research design so that we could gather objective data with which to test the elements of the approach.

We would also be more sensitive to the identification of and significance of individual variables affecting the condition of obesity so that we could deal more effectively with these. One of these significant variables is the obese adolescent's family situation. We felt that more sharing with and involvement of the parents in the program's goals would help them to function in a supportive way with the adolescent. The fact that an adolescent girl spends most of her time in a particular home environment with its multiple significant forces, that she is still quite dependent on her parents for support, and that her mother often does the cooking are important factors to consider if a treatment program is to be successful.

We have no data to support the procedure of separation of boys and girls in an obesity group. We can only say that it seemed easier to deal only with girls. For example, we could not have done the grooming session as we did if we had included boys. However, it might be helpful in future attempts to try to run the group with both boys and girls.

Lastly, we would select the group more carefully in order to have more homogeneity in terms of developmental maturity. Chronologic age is a poor criterion to use in judging maturity. It is also important to remember that we cannot group all adolescents together and label them as alike; there are vast individual differences within this age group. We would therefore select girls who demonstrated similar concerns, needs, and interests; a high degree of internal motivation; and an ability to set realistic goals for weight loss. We found that the more mature girls in our group were more responsive, more interested, and better able to follow through, and thus success was favored.

## Summary

We feel that it is essential to intervene during adolescence in dealing with the problem of obesity, for at this time the individual is most concerned about the condition and capable of altering it. Also, if the problem is ignored past this crucial time, it will have lasting negative effects on the individual and will probably be essentially untreatable.

In our opinion, use of the group approach is of considerable importance in dealing with this problem because of the adolescent's great reliance on peer support. We also feel that the approach used should be aimed primarily at breaking the vicious cycle of negative psychosocial perpetuating factors and not just narrowly focused upon either diet or activity alone. That is, not merely the obesity, but the total adolescent—her psychologic and social needs, characteristics, and worries, and her environmental background—must be taken into consideration if the approach is to be effective.

Finally, we consider long-term continuity with the same respected role model to be essential in building a therapeutic relationship which ultimately should be helpful in altering this chronic problem of obesity.

## REFERENCES

1.  Hammar ST: Adolescence. In Baker GT (ed): Obesity in Pediatric Practice. Report of the Second Ross Roundtable, Feb 1971, p 17
2.  Stunkard A: Psychologic factors. In Baker GT (ed): Obesity in Pediatric Practice. Report of the Second Ross Roundtable, Feb 1971, p 32
3.  Vastbinder EE: The treatment of adolescent obesity: exploration of method of treatment. Master's thesis, Ohio State U, 1967
4.  Gallagher JR: Medical Care of the Adolescent. New York: Appleton, 1960, p 139

5.  Spargo JA, et al: Adolescent obesity. Nutrition Today 1:4, Dec 1966, p 9
6.  Daniel WA, Jr: The Adolescent Patient. St Louis, Mosby, 1970, p 99
7.  Mayer J: Obesity in childhood and adolescence. Med Clin North Am 48:5, Sept 1964, p 1355
8.  Beland IT: Clinical Nursing: Pathophysiological and Psychosocial Approaches. New York: Macmillan, 1973, p 551
9.  Smart MA, Smart RC: Children: Development and Relationships. New York, Macmillan, 1967, p 438
10. Sherman L: Psychology of physical illness in adolescents. Pediatr Clin North Am 7:1, Feb 1960, p 86
11. Schonfeld WA: Body-image in adolescents: a psychiatric concept for the pediatrician. Pediatrics, May 1963, p 849
12. Hammar ST: An interdisciplinary study of adolescent obesity. J Pediatr 80:3, March 1972, pp 377, 378
13. Langdell JI: A psychiatric approach to obesity in childhood and adolescence. In Szurek SA (ed): Psychosomatic Disorders and Mental Retardation. Palo Alto, Science and Behavior Books, 1968
14. Stanley EJ, et al: Overcoming obesity in adolescents: a description of a promising endeavor to improve management. Clin Pediatr, Jan 1970, pp 33, 34
15. Bruch H: Psychological aspects of obesity. Bordens Rev Nutr Res 19:4, July–August 1958, pp 69, 70
16. Ohlsen M: Group Counseling. New York, Holt, 1970, p 101
17. Berkovitz IH: On growing a group: some thoughts on structure, process, and setting. In Berkovitz IH (ed): Adolescents Grow in Groups. New York: Brunner/Mazel, 1972, p 8
18. Schutz W: Joy: Expanding Human Awareness. New York, Grove, 1967, p 11

BIBLIOGRAPHY

Bruch H: Psychological aspects of obesity. Borden's Rev Nutr Res 19:4, July–August 1958
Hammar ST: Adolescence. In Baker GT (ed): Obesity in Pediatric Practice, Report of the Second Ross Roundtable, Feb 1971
Hammar ST, et al: An interdisciplinary study of adolescent obesity. J Pediatr 80:3, Mar 1972
Langdell JI: A psychiatric approach to obesity in childhood and adolescence. In Szurek SA (ed): Psychosomatic Disorders and Mental Retardation. Palo Alto, Science and Behavior Books, 1968
Mayer J: Obesity in childhood and adolescence. Med Clin North Am 48:5, Sept 1964
Ohlsen M: Group Counseling. New York, Holt, 1970

Schonfeld WA: Body-image in adolescents: A psychiatric concept for the pediatrician. Pediatrics, May 1963

Schutz W: Joy: Expanding Human Awareness. New York, Grove, 1967

Smart MS, Smart RC: Children: Development and Relationships. New York, Macmillan, 1967

Spargo JA, et al: Adolescent obesity. Nutrition Today 1:4, Dec 1966

Stanley EJ, et al: Overcoming obesity in adolescents. A description of a promising endeavor to improve management. Clin Pediatr, Jan 1970

Stunkard A: Psychologic factors. Obesity in Pediatric Practice, Report of the Second Ross Roundtable, Feb 1971

Vastbinder EE: Exploration of method of treatment. The treatment of adolescent obesity. Master's thesis, Ohio State U, 1967

# 6
# Venereal Disease in the Adolescent

FRANCIS W. EBERLY

The alarming increase in venereal disease (VD) among young people presents a critical challenge to the nurse and other health practitioners caring for the adolescent. Possibly as many as three or four out of every one hundred 15- to 19-year-olds in the United States will contract gonorrhea this year, and as many as six or seven out of every one hundred 20- to 24-year-olds.

The adolescent who recognizes he has contracted a venereal disease is involved with many conflicting and confusing feelings: What do I do now, where do I go for help, what will happen if my parents find out? The careless, naive, or uninformed teenager presents other challenges to the nursing and medical profession. How can proper educational, medical, and counseling services be established to assist these young people who ignorantly experiment with their newfound sexual prowess? This chapter will detail the steady increase in the rate of VD in the adolescent population, offer a general review of the major venereal

109

diseases encountered in clinical practice, and suggest some epidemiologic and counseling attitudes that may be helpful to the nurse involved in the care of young people.

The term "venereal" comes from the name of the goddess Venus, the mother of Cupid in Roman mythology. It refers to anything relating to intimate expressions of affection between two persons. Venereal diseases are diseases transmitted between two members of the same or opposite sex through intimate, direct bodily contact. Venereal disease germs are not transmitted, as many other bacterial and viral infections are, by air or by contact with contaminated eating utensils or toilet seats.

In the United States five venereal diseases are by law considered reportable: gonorrhea, syphilis, chancroid, lymphogranuloma venereum, and granuloma inguinale. The last three are considered minor venereal diseases as they constitute less than one percent of the total number of cases of venereal diseases reported. A number of other sexually transmitted diseases and infestations are emerging as significant conditions among our youth and college-age adults. These conditions will be briefly discussed.

## INCIDENCE OF VENEREAL DISEASE IN ADOLESCENTS AND YOUNG ADULTS

The incidence of gonorrhea in the United States is greater than that of any other communicable disease requiring treatment (Fig. 1). In the 1960s the attack rate of gonorrhea began a steady unrelenting climb to the record high rate in 1973 of 392.2 cases per 100,000 in the general population. In fiscal year 1973, 809,681 cases of gonorrhea were reported to local health departments in the United States.[1] Figure 2 graphically illustrates the number of reported cases of gonorrhea in the United States in the past 22 years. In the six-year span from 1966 to 1972 the number of reported cases of gonorrhea increased 106 percent. In the calendar

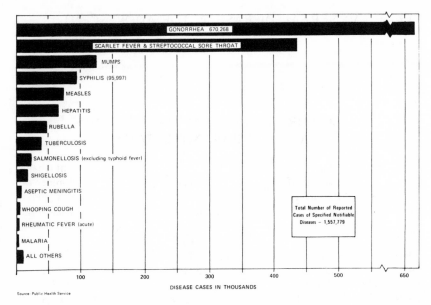

FIG. 1. Number of reported cases of communicable diseases in the United States in 1971. (Courtesy of Public Health Service.)

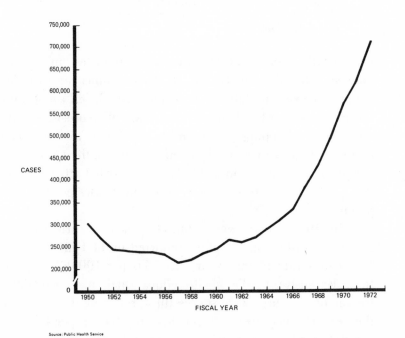

FIG. 2. Reported cases of gonorrhea in the United States from 1950 to 1972.

Table 1

### GONORRHEA: MORBIDITY IN ADOLESCENTS, AGE 15 TO 19 IN UNITED STATES*

| Year | Number of Reported Cases | Rate per 100,000 Population | Percent Change in Number of Cases from Previous Year |
|------|--------------------------|-----------------------------|------------------------------------------------------|
| 1956 | 45,161 | 415.7 | — |
| 1966 | 76,032 | 436.1 | — |
| 1967 | 91,390 | 531.0 | +20.2 |
| 1968 | 108,405 | 610.6 | +18.6 |
| 1969 | 129,071 | 712.5 | +18.8 |
| 1970 | 147,942 | 808.6 | +14.6 |
| 1971 | 171,581 | 887.3 | +16.0 |
| 1972 | 204,635 | 1,035.4 | +19.2 |

*Courtesy of the U.S. Public Health Service*

year 1972, over 515,000 cases were reported in youths between the ages of 15 to 24. This number of cases of gonorrhea exceeded all the reported cases in *all* age groups for mumps, measles, hepatitis, rubella, tuberculosis, aseptic meningitis, whooping cough, and acute rheumatic fever. The number of cases of gonorrhea reported in youths 15 to 19 in recent years is shown in Table 1. The reported attack rate in the 15 to 19 age group is now over 1,000 cases per 100,000 population.

In 1947, there were 106,539 cases of primary and secondary (infectious) syphilis reported in the United States. The attack rate in that year was 75.6 per 100,000 population. Extensive public health educational, diagnostic, and treatment measures were successful in reducing this rate over the next 10 years to an all time low of 3.8 cases per 100,000 population. Table 2 shows the increase, with a brief decline in the late 1960s, in the number of reported cases of infectious syphilis over the past 11 years.

Table 2

## PRIMARY AND SECONDARY SYPHILIS:
## UNITED STATES*

| Year | Number of Reported Cases | Rate per 100,000 Population | Percent Change in Number of Cases from Previous Year |
|------|-----|-----|-----|
| 1957 | 6,251 | 3.8 | — |
| 1963 | 22,045 | 11.9 | + 9.8 |
| 1964 | 22,733 | 12.1 | + 3.1 |
| 1965 | 23,250 | 12.3 | + 2.3 |
| 1966 | 22,473 | 11.6 | − 3.3 |
| 1967 | 21,090 | 10.8 | − 6.1 |
| 1968 | 20,182 | 10.3 | − 4.3 |
| 1969 | 18,679 | 9.3 | − 7.4 |
| 1970 | 20,186 | 10.0 | + 8.1 |
| 1971 | 23,336 | 11.5 | +15.6 |
| 1972 | 24,000 | 11.7 | + 2.8 |
| 1973 | 25,080 | 12.1 | + 9.5 |

*Courtesy of the U.S. Public Health Service

The attack rate for adolescents age 15 to 19 for syphilis in 1972 was 20.4 per 100,000, and 42.1 cases per 100,000 population in 20- to 24-year-old youths, nearly four times the national rate.[1]

The Public Health Service estimates that the reported figures for venereal disease represent only the "tip of the iceberg." Possibly as many as three to four times this number of cases of VD are contracted each year but are not reported. The vast reservoir of asymptomatic, undiagnosed female carriers of gonorrhea presents a serious public health problem. Furthermore, the ease with which the young male is diagnosed as having gonorrhea, ie, marked early clinical symptoms, simple office procedure of staining urethral discharge to confirm diagnosis, and lack of formal laboratory culture reports which by law must be reported to health departments, leads to significant underreporting of gonorrhea in the male.

## Factors Contributing to Increase of Venereal Disease in Adolescents

Dr. Kampmeier of Vanderbilt, in a classic article entitled "Venereal Disease in the Teenager," states:

The increase in teenage non-marital sexual experience has been documented repeatedly in terms of illegitimate births, criminal abortions, and the rising incidence of venereal disease. Despite claims that the "sexual revolution" is largely a matter of freer verbalization and news media exaggeration, the facts point to earlier sexual activities among teenagers in heterosexual coitus, homosexuality, and non-coital heterosexual experimentation.[2]

Dr. Kampmeier cites a World Health Organization report[3] which concluded that the following factors have a role in the increasing rate of venereal disease: (1) "ignorance of the nature and meaning of sex and of the dangers of abuse of sexual functions"; (2) "the decline in religious faith;" (3) "the emancipation of woman"; (4) "the lack of discipline in home life and of parental supervision"; (5) "the failure of fear as a deterrent"; (6) "the emphasis on sexuality in books, plays, and films, on television, and in advertisements"; (7) "misinterpretation of psychologic teaching"; (8) "earlier physical development." While all might not agree as to the relative importance of each of these causes, the social situation that they indicate in the United States has not changed since this 1965 report.

The pseudosophisticated adolescent who engages in promiscuous sexual relations presents an appalling unconcern about acquiring VD. The "experienced" male teenager can readily obtain treatment for his repeated attacks of gonorrhea. He has little knowledge of possible complications of the disease and no appreciation for preventive measures.

The furor in the late 1960s over "sex education" in the schools led many school boards to discontinue or significantly alter sound educational programs of health education and responsible human sexuality. Teenagers of today no longer accept the moral "Thou shall nots" of the Judeo-Christian ethic without wanting to know the psychologic and interpersonal reasons behind these "old fashioned" black-and-white rules.

Celia Deschin, writing in the American Journal of Nursing,[4] states, "Given the widespread permissiveness as regards pre-marital sex relations and an emphasis on sexuality divorced from interpersonal relationships and responsibility, a concept of sex has been developing that is biological rather than biological and social, a concept that has not been challenged by the adult world to the point where the adolescent would know what is the desired standard to which he is expected to adhere. It is not surprising that sex becomes merely a release of physiological tension, an index of masculine prowess or of feminine popularity, or even a commodity with which to buy dates, clothes, friendship, affection, or other lacks in life."

## Symptomatology and Management of Sexually Transmitted Diseases

### GONORRHEA

Gonorrhea, also known in the streets as "clap," "strain," "GC," "the dose," or "the drip," is caused by a gram-negative diplococcus, the bacterium *Neisseria gonorrhoeae*. The organism penetrates the lining of the urethra in the male and commonly affects the lower genitourinary tract. Symptoms in the male can occur as soon as one day following exposure or as late as three or four weeks following sexual contact. The mean incubation period for males is three to five days.[5]

The diagnosis of acute gonorrhea in the male presents little or no difficulty. Over 90 percent of males who contract the infection will develop urinary frequency followed by a mucoid urethral discharge which progresses in a matter of hours to a purulent yellow discharge accompanied by marked dysuria. These symptoms usually lead the adolescent to some type of medical attention, yet all too often the youth will resort to self-treatment with "leftover pills" or hope that he will get better on his own. The infection remains localized to the anterior urethra for the first two weeks or so and then spreads back to the prostate and the seminal vesicles. There it may smoulder or flare up into painful epididymitis.

Laboratory confirmation of the diagnosis of gonorrhea in the male is rapidly accomplished by a gram stain of the urethral discharge. If no discharge is easily expressed, a urethro-genital swab is inserted into the urethra and a gentle scraping of the wall of the urethra is smeared onto a slide and stained. The infecting organisms are easily identified as gram-negative intracellular diplococci in the smears. This type of organism does not normally inhabit the male genitourinary tract in contrast to the findings in smears from the female genital tract. Early in the disease in the male, the GC organisms may be seen only outside the pus cell (poly-morphonuclear cell) and often the pus cells are fragmented. If the youth has taken an antibiotic shortly before the smear examination, the gonococci may appear swollen and dis-torted, making the diagnosis more difficult. If no intracellular diplococci are seen on a smear at the initial visit a urethral culture obtained with a wire loop should be planted and incubated on Thayer-Martin culture media.

In the female it is difficult, if not impossible, to know when symptoms of gonorrhea first begin. The vast majority of women remain asymptomatic of the disease and continue to be highly infective transmitters of GC for many months. Some commercial serologic tests are now available, yet the firm diagnosis must be made by cervical and rectal cultures obtained during a pelvic examination. Recent reports have indicated a surprisingly high incidence of positive gonococcal cultures from the rectum of asymptomatic women.[6, 7]

Infection of the rectum in women is usually secondary to genital infection spreading by accidental self-inoculation to the rectum, but may also occur as a result of anal intercourse. The finding of rectal gonorrhea in the male is invariably a consequence of homosexual practices.[8]

A pelvic examination and appropriate cultures for gonorrhea should never be delayed in a young woman who is a possible gonorrhea contact, or who has a recently acquired vaginal discharge, just because she is menstruating. There is a greater chance of culturing the gonococci during menstruation, and delay in diagnosis may result in infection spreading to the upper genital tract or allow a potentially infected person to spread the infection further.

*Complications of Gonorrhea.* The major early stage complications of untreated gonorrhea in women are as follows:

1. Ascending upper genital tract inflammation is known as acute pelvic inflammatory disease (PID). Typically, patients with acute PID present with chills, fever, severe bilateral lower abdominal pain, and rebound tenderness caused by acute purulent salpingitis and pelvic peritonitis. Adequate treatment with appropriate antibiotics can usually be accomplished without hospitalization. Repeated bouts of inflammatory disease leading to abscess formation require hospital care and a combination of antibiotics given parenterally.

2. Gonococcal arthritis, the most common cause of infectious arthritis, occurs five times more frequently in the female than in the male.[9] Females are much more susceptible during menstruation and pregnancy. The arthritis usually involves several joints, the most common being the wrist, knee, and ankle. The bacteremic phase of the disease is often accompanied by a hemorrhagic or pustular rash of the extremities. The diagnosis is confirmed by isolating the

gonococcus in cultures from synovial fluid but this is possible in only about 25 percent of the cases.

The disease must be suspected on clinical grounds and appropriate cultures taken from the endocervical canal and rectum. Hospital care is usually necessary in the management of gonococcal arthritis. Effective treatment includes large doses of parenteral penicillin, 10 to 20 million units per day for 7 to 10 days. Response is usually evident within 48 hours and all manifestations disappear usually within 7 to 10 days.

3. Perihepatitis, a rare syndrome resembling acute cholecystitis or perforated peptic ulcer, has until recently been seen only in women. The spread of the gonococcus from the open fallopian tubes occurred most likely by way of the pelvic lymphatics to the capsule of the liver to form adhesions. The report of this syndrome occurring in the male[10] has led to the belief that the organism may be spread by other lymphatic systems or is blood borne.

4. Other life threatening complications of acute gonorrhea include carditis, septicemia, and meningitis.

*Treatment of Gonorrhea.* The following treatment schedule for uncomplicated gonococcal infections of the urethra, cervix, pharynx, and rectum has been recently recommended by the Center for Disease Control in Atlanta, Georgia:

Parenteral    — Aqueous procaine penicillin G 4.8 million units given intramuscularly with 1.0 gram probenecid by mouth (preferably given at least 30 minutes prior to injection)

Oral    — Ampicillin 3.5 grams by mouth with 1.0 gram probenecid by mouth (may be given simultaneously)

Parenteral* — Spectinomycin 2.0 grams intramuscularly in males, 4.0 grams intramuscularly in females

Oral* — Tetracycline HCL 1.5 grams by mouth stat, then 0.5 grams by mouth qid for 4 days (total 9.5 grams)

*For patients in whom penicillin is contraindicated (may include allergy to penicillin, asthma, hay fever, etc.) or in whom penicillin or ampicillin has been ineffective.*

It must be emphasized that only the parenteral administration of aqueous procaine penicillin in the above dosage has been recently shown to be also almost 100 percent effective in aborting incubating syphilis.[11]

All other forms of treatment, including ampicillin, spectinomycin, tetracycline and its derivatives, require monthly VDRL serology examination for four months after initial treatment of gonorrhea to detect the possible development of infectious syphilis acquired at the time of exposure to gonorrhea and which may have been masked by treatment.

SYPHILIS

Syphilis, also called *lues* from the Latin word meaning "the plague," is caused by the delicate spirochete *Treponema pallidum*. The organism requires a warm, moist environment for survival and is transmitted by intimate bodily contact. Following an incubation period of approximately 9 to 90 days after exposure (average three weeks) the lesion of primary syphilis appears at the site of infection as an indurated painless ulcer, usually a single lesion. The chancre occurs on the genitalia, rectum, lips, or on the mucosal lining of the mouth. In the female the site of penetration of the spirochete is often the cervix and the resulting painless chancre remains unrecognized. If this primary stage of syphilis remains unrecognized and untreated the chancre may last from 3 to 12 weeks and then heal spontaneously.

After approximately six weeks to six months following the primary stage the patient develops the highly infectious stage of secondary syphilis. Symptoms of secondary lues include maculopapular eruptions, commonly on the palms and soles, generalized measles-like rash over the body, mucous patches found in the mouth, rectum, and vagina, and patchy alopecia. Moist, flat, wartlike lesions called condylomata lata can appear in the anogenital and other moist areas of the body. They must be distinguished from the common viral condition called genital warts or condylomata accuminata.

Systemic symptoms of fever, malaise, generalized lymphadenopathy, headache, sore throat, and clinical findings of hepatitis or renal disease can occur during this stage of syphilis. Clinicians of a few generations ago properly dubbed syphilis as the "great imitator."

The positive diagnosis of syphilis in the primary stage of the chancre requires a special dark-field microscopic examination of serum obtained from the base of the lesion. The characteristic motion of the coiled spirochete of *T. pallidum* confirms the diagnosis. This test has two distinct disadvantages:

1. The dark-field microscope must be available near the examining room when appropriate specimens are obtained from the patient.
2. Specimens taken from a lesion of the mucous lining of the mouth may contain normal floral spirochetes which are indistinguishable from the infecting organism *T. pallidum,* leading to a false positive diagnosis.

Most physicians do not have ready access to a dark-field microscope. In some communities, this examination can only be done at the local health department. A new examination procedure, not yet commercially available, is the fluorescent antibody dark-field exam (FADF). This test will allow the physician to mail a specimen to a central laboratory for positive diagnosis.

The diagnosis of the infectious stage of syphilis is most often made by a positive serologic test. It must be remembered that it takes several weeks to develop the appropriate antibodies to the germ before serologic tests are reactive. A significant number of patients have a positive serologic test for syphilis when the primary chancre first appears. However, a negative serologic test in the presence of a suspicious lesion does not rule out the diagnosis of primary syphilis.

The VDRL (Venereal Disease Research Laboratory) test is the serologic test of choice in the screening of patients for syphilis and in the follow-up of patients treated for the disease. It is cheap, easy to do, rapid, and, when the test is positive in a significant titer, practically confirms the diagnosis. The disadvantages of this test are that it is not always specific or sensitive enough to detect early disease, and several other disease states, narcotics addiction, and even recent smallpox vaccination can cause a biologic false positive test (BFP).

The FTA-ABS (Fluorescent Treponema Antibody Absorbed) test offers several advantages over the VDRL. It is more specific and becomes positive earlier in the primary stage of syphilis than the VDRL. Some patients with increased or abnormal serum globulins will give a biologic false positive reaction to the test but this is infrequent.[12] The test is difficult to perform, not available everywhere, and remains positive after treatment, thus rendering it useless in evaluating effective therapy of active disease.

*Complications of Syphilis.*   If the infectious stage of secondary syphilis remains untreated the lesions heal spontaneously in approximately one to three months and the patient enters the latent or tertiary stage of the disease. For the next four years (early latent stage) the patient is potentially infectious. (The severe, life-threatening complications of late syphilis involving the cardiovascular and neurologic systems will not be described.)

*Treatment of Primary and Secondary Syphilis.*   Penicillin is the drug of choice for the treatment of all stages of syphilis in the nonallergenic patient. No evidence has emerged to indicate the development of resistance to penicillin by the infecting spirochete.

The following treatment schedule for infectious syphilis is recommended by CDC:[13]

Primary and Secondary Syphilis

℞:  Benzathine penicillin G—Total dosage: 2.4 million units (1.2 million units in each buttock) by intramuscular injection

or:  Procaine penicillin G in oil with aluminum monostearate (PAM)—Total dosage: 4.8 million units (2.4 million units at first session, as above, and 1.2 million units at each of the two subsequent injections, 3 days apart)

or:  Aqueous procaine penicillin G—Total dosage 4.8 million units (600,000 units daily for 8 days)

For patients allergic to penicillin: Tetracycline (total dose 30 gm) 500 mg orally four times a day for 15 days

For pregnant patients allergic to penicillin: Erythromycin (total dose 40 gm) 500 mg orally four times a day for 20 days

Following treatment of infectious syphilis the patient must be followed with a repeat physical examination and repeat VDRL at 1, 3, 6, 9, 12, 18, and 24 months. The lesions should not reappear and the VDRL should continue to diminish. At the end of two years, the VDRL should be seronegative or remain serofast at a low titer. A return of the lesions of primary or secondary syphilis, or a rise in titer of over two dilutions, indicates relapse or reinfection and must be retreated with double the dose of antibiotics recommended for infectious syphilis.[14]

## The Minor Reportable Venereal Diseases

*Chancroid* is caused by a gram-negative bacillus which after an incubation period of from two to five days produces painful ulcers and enlarged suppurative inguinal nodes called "bubos." The diagnosis can be made by identifying the bacteria from the ulcers or lymph glands by smear or culture.

Over 50 percent of the less than 2,000 cases each year are reported from the South Atlantic States.

*Lymphogranuloma venereum*, as the name implies, is a disease of the inguinal and femoral lymph glands which if untreated leads to suppuration and scarring of superficial and deep pelvic lymph channels. The causative agent is a virus, and treatment with tetracycline or sulfonamides over several weeks may be effective.

*Granuloma inguinale*, a bacterial disease producing lesions in the groin, perineum, or genitals, may cause very extensive red, raised, velvety granulomatous lesions which bleed easily. The characteristic finding of Donovan bodies in the mononuclear cells confirms the diagnosis. Tetracycline, 2 grams per day for three weeks, is effective but follow-up is important as relapses do occur. Over the past 10 years, less than 200 cases per year have been reported in the United States.[15]

## Other Sexually Transmitted Diseases

### TRICHOMONIASIS

The parasite *Trichomonas vaginalis* may produce a copious, frothy, greenish-yellow vaginal discharge in adolescent girls and is the cause of some cases of urethritis in the male. The infection is sexually transmitted and if both partners are not treated simultaneously, the infection may "ping-pong" back and forth.

The treatment of trichomoniasis of the genital tract of both sexual partners is with the drug metronidazole (Flagyl®). The adolescent dose for girls is the same as for the adult (one tablet three times a day by mouth after meals for 10 days). If the adolescent girl has only one sexual partner she must be told that she likely received the infection from her asymptomatic consort and that, if he is not treated, he may well reinfect her if relations are continued. The dosage for the male is one tablet by mouth twice a day for ten days.

Trichomonas vaginitis, while one of the commonest causes of leukorrhea in adolescents, is also a common accompanying disease in girls with gonorrhea. Thus the finding of the pear-shaped, wriggling protozoa in the wet mount should not lull one into the belief that only one disease is present. Appropriate cultures for GC must also be obtained.

## HEMOPHILUS VAGINITIS

The organism *Hemophilus vaginalis* is a short, rod-shaped, gram-negative bacillus and is essentially the only cause of bacterial vaginitis in the adolescent and the adult other than the gonococcus. The infection causes a gray, white, homogeneous, malodorous discharge which is not as profuse or watery as that seen in trichomonal vaginitis, nor does it produce the red, inflamed vulvar and vaginal irritation as seen in monilial infection. Microscopic examination of the wet mount saline slide shows the diagnostic "clue cells"— superficial vaginal epithelial cells with a stippled or granulated look due to the masses of *H. vaginalis* bacteria on the cell surface. In the gram stain of the vaginal secretions, only a few pus cells are seen, the Doderlein bacilli (gram-positive lactobacilli) are usually absent, and clumps of the small gram-negative rods of *H. vaginalis* are seen. Culture of the organism is difficult but Casmen's blood agar base (Difco®) incubated under reduced oxygen tension is an appropriate medium.

Treatment with Terramycin® vaginal suppositories nightly for 10 days is effective but may cause an overgrowth of candida (monilia). Oral ampicillin, 500 mg every six hours for five days, has been recommended for both sexual partners. It is thought that 25 percent of females with trichomoniasis also have a hemophilus infection.[16]

## GENITAL HERPES

Herpetic vulvitis caused by herpes simplex virus, type 2, formerly considered to be a rare cause of vulvar irritation, is rapidly becoming a significant infection in adolescent girls.[16] Grouped, clear vesicles 1 to 5 mm in diameter are formed on the vulva and surrounding skin of the perineum. The vesicles rapidly break down into small confluent ulcers and secondary bacterial infection with tissue necrosis is common. Lesions around the urethral opening may cause dysuria without urinary frequency. Laboratory examination is required to confirm the diagnosis of herpes genitalis but treatment of herpetic ulcerations is unsatisfactory as there are no specific remedies yet available for recurrent attacks.

## PEDICULOSIS PUBIS

Crab lice, like gonorrhea, are becoming an ever increasing medical problem among young people who have intimate close bodily contact. The parasite, a tiny 1 mm, six-clawed louse is usually transmitted from person to person but can also be transmitted through interchange of contaminated blankets or clothing, and even may be acquired from infested toilet seats and beds. Crab lice should be suspected when the patient complains of pubic or vulvar itching. A careful examination of the pubic hair area under a magnifying glass and bright light will reveal the movement of one or two of the lice. Treatment consists of a shampoo of the infected area with 1 percent gamma-benzine hexachloride (Kwell®). The treatment should be repeated 7 to 10 days later to remove any nits (eggs) which have hatched into adult lice. All

contaminated clothing should be thoroughly washed or dry
cleaned.

## Toward Abatement of Venereal Disease in Adolescents

### THROUGH EDUCATION

Ten years ago the writers of the 1963 Joint Statement were
hopeful about prospects for the future control of venereal
disease in teenagers. "The widespread awakening to the
seriousness of the VD problem in their own jurisdictions by
city and state health officers; the increasing awareness
demonstrated by private practicing physicians in their role in
venereal disease control and the recent wide publicity given
by the mass media exposing the extent and character of the
problem to the public, all add up to one word—progress."
The hope was also expressed that enough interest would be
generated among the public and the medical profession to
develop a twofold approach to VD control—increased
educational efforts and the promotion of physician—health
department cooperation—to reach the American teenager
who contracts VD.[17]
 This optimistic hope of a decade ago has been shattered
by present-day facts. In only the past five years, the attack
rate of gonorrhea among 15- to 19-year-olds has doubled. In
the next ten years the present-day population of 15-year-old
boys and girls in the United States (approximately 4 million)
will inevitably contract and share between 3 and 4 million
cases of gonorrhea and syphilis even if the attack rate does
*not* increase. There are no other disease states that will affect
so many young people over a 10-year period, and that carry
such potential consequences, that have received less public
attention.
 Today's young people do not know nearly as much as
they should, or as much as they think they know, about the
venereal diseases. Many middle schools and high schools are

not teaching anything about the diseases, as they have either attempted to ignore the serious reality of the epidemic or have been subjected to parental objection to the controversial aspect of teaching "sex education." In 1971, 73 percent of the junior and senior high schools included venereal disease information in their curriculum. In the following year, replies to the Joint Statement questionnaire indicated that schools in only 60 percent of the counties and cities included such information. Comments from health officers suggested that in some areas there was significant opposition to venereal disease information in the schools:

> A formal and structured VD information and educational program has now lapsed in the public school system. We are informed that there has been parental resistance and objection expressly over sex information and education. (A city in Florida)

> State Legislature moratorium on sex education in effect. This limits VD education for fear of violating moratorium. (A city in Louisiana)[1]

Venereal disease education in secondary schools must not become entangled with the issue of "sex education," and all the accompanying morality hang-ups which create road blocks to teaching efforts. Gonorrhea is the leading infectious, *communicable* disease which requires treatment that will likely affect our youth. VD education must be a significant part of the curriculum on *communicable* diseases. The school nurse or the regular classroom teacher of science or health must be the person to instruct our youth that venereal diseases do exist, that they are epidemic, that some students might be affected by them, and that they can and must do something about them.

In some places, young people themselves have taken on the responsibility for educating their peers about VD. In Philadelphia, for example, the Community Service Corps of the Philadelphia Archdiocese maintains "Operation Venus," a group of seventy-five volunteers who are providing an intensive VD education program aimed at the city's youth. The young people, carefully trained by health officials, maintain a speakers' bureau, operate a VD "hot line," make arrangements for the rapid, confidential diagnosis and treatment of any youth who thinks he may be infected, and even provides immediate transportation to clinics or to offices of volunteer doctors for evaluation. The adult sponsorship of such programs by school nurses, physicians, and local PTA organizations could give great impetus to similar programs around the country. Today's students do not want to be "preached at" or given half-truths about venereal disease. They deserve the attention of interested professional people who can discuss sensitive subjects with them in a nonjudgmental yet straightforward fashion.

In this era of sexual frankness, it is not too much to ask of the youth with venereal disease to urge their sexual contacts to seek medical care promptly. The school or clinic nurse can help the adolescent understand that the treatment of VD in most states can be accomplished without parental knowledge or consent. If the problems of the infected youth and his contacts are presented seriously, candidly, and confidentially the adolescent will invariably cooperate.

## REFERENCES

1. Today's VD Control Problem—1974. American Social Health Association, New York, N.Y.
2. Kampmeier RH: Venereal disease in the teenager. Medical Aspects of Human Sexuality, March 1968
3. King A: Venereal disease among young people—report of a WHO expert committee on the health problems of adolescence. WHO Chronicle 19:144, 1965
4. Deschin CS: VD and adolescent personality. Am J Nurs 63:58, 1963
5. Fiumara NJ: Diagnosis and treatment of gonorrhea. Clin Med 74:29, 1967

6. Schmale JD, Martin JE Jr., Domesick G: Observations on the cultural diagnosis of gonorrhea in women. JAMA 210:312–314, 1969
7. Schroeter AL, Reynolds G: The rectal culture as a test of cure of gonorrhea in the female. J Infect Dis 125:499, 1972
8. Owen RL, Hill JL: Gonorrhea in homosexual men. JAMA 220:1315, 1972
9. Cooke CL, Owen DS Jr., Irby R, Toone E: Gonococcal arthritis. JAMA 217:204, 1971
10. Kimball MW, Knee S: Gonococcal perihepatitis in the male. N Eng J Med 282:1082, 1970
11. Schroeter AL, Turner RH, Lucas JB, Brown WJ: Therapy for incubating syphilis. JAMA 218:711, 1971
12. Mackey DM, Price EV, Knox JM, Scotti A: Specificity of the FTA-ABS test for syphilis. JAMA 207:1683, 1969
13. Venereal Disease Program, Center for Disease Control—Syphilis: A Symposium. U.S. Public Health Service Publication No. 1660, 1968
14. Drusin LM: The diagnosis and treatment of infectious syphilis. Med Clin North Am 56:1161, Sept 1972
15. VD Fact Sheet 1972. U.S. Department of Health, Education and Welfare Public Health Service
16. Altcher A: Adolescent vulvovaginitis. Pediatr Clin North Am 19:735, August 1972
17. Today's VD Control Problem—1963. New York, American Social Health Association

# 7

# Drug Abuse in Adolescence

JOHN N. STEPHENSON

Drug abuse as with most other organic and psychologic disorders is not unique to adolescence. In fact, a far more serious problem exists among our adult population with its between five and ten million alcoholics. Nevertheless, our youth today are more seriously involved with drug abuse than ever before. Consequently, an adolescent's presenting complaint may very well center around a drug-related issue. It is often the nurse, in her multiple professional capacities, who initially must face this issue. How one views youthful drug abuse and how one responds accordingly under conditions of a drug-induced crisis may at times prove to be a vital issue in the ultimate outcome for the adolescent.

A multitude of surveys have been done concerning the nonmedical use of drugs.[1-5] One of the more recent consisted of a survey of 15,634 students in grades 6 through 12 living in Anchorage, Alaska in 1971.[5] The findings of this survey demonstrate the pervasive use of numerous chemicals and how the use of drugs has progressively involved younger and younger age groups. Alcohol, tobacco, marijuana, solvents, nonprescription stimulants, and hashish were the most commonly reported drugs for all students. Any drug with mind-altering properties has been utilized to meet the various emotional needs of the adolescent. However, heavy use of amphetamines, hallucinogens, and especially heroin was not found in this survey by virtue of the fact that users have already dropped out of school. The physical and psychologic dependency on "hard" drugs compels the addict to devote most of his energy toward procurement of the necessary dosage.

## WHY YOUTHFUL DRUG ABUSE?

In a report by the Committee on Youth of the American Academy of Pediatrics, a personal communication of Graham Blaine, former Chief of Psychiatry in the Student Health Services at Harvard, has summarized some of the forces that influence boys and girls of junior high and high school age in the abuse of drugs. Dr. Blaine felt that youths take drugs to prove their courage by indulging in risk-taking; act out their rebellion and hostility toward authority; facilitate sexual desires and performance; elevate themselves from loneliness and provide an emotional experience; attempt to find the meaning of life.[6] Very broadly, drug abuse can be described as an effort by individuals to feel differently than they do.

Dr. Blaine's explanation for drug abuse can most aptly be applied to the middle-adolescent period. The adoption of the peer group's ideas and values with respect to dress, language, music, and dance stabilizes the adolescent identity as the individual further separates himself from his family. But this very conformity may lead to group behavioral experimentation with drugs. This particular form of drug abuse, while risky from a legal and potential-accident point of view, is less precarious than solo drug abuse in this age group. For lack of friends, poor peer group ties, and sexual promiscuity also portray an emotionally unhealthy adolescent in whom drug abuse may prove disastrous.

It is not surprising to find that, with increasing availability of drugs, the emerging and vulnerable adolescent in the sixth and seventh grades is increasingly found to be experimenting with them. This age perhaps more than any other finds itself in a psychologic void. At this point the youth are neither dependently tied to parents nor accepted into the peer group. The rejection of parental values and the independent-dependent struggle may lead to mood swings, depression, boredom, periodic regressive retreats into childhood and mild antisocial behavior.[7] School failure, school dropout, and frequent solo drug use are pathologic complications of early adolescence. As is apparent, solo drug abuse is only one expression of an adolescent in trouble. However, a flight from reality via drug abuse may seriously compromise an adolescent's emotional development.

One might expect that increasing maturity associated with late adolescence would see a lessening of drug abuse. The Anchorage, Alaska, school survey does not support this premise but instead demonstrates a steady increase in use with advancing age through the junior high and high school years.[5]

Tec studied some aspects of the relationship of high school status and differential involvement with marijuana in 1,704 teenage boys and girls enrolled in the only high school of a well-to-do New York suburban community.[8] He concludes that there is a negative association between satisfaction with formal aspects of school and marijuana use. The less satisfied and involved a high school student is, the more likely he is to smoke marijuana with regularity and the less likely he is never to have had any experience with this drug. The more involved and committed a youngster is to the formal aspects of the educational system, the less likely he is to use marijuana with regularity. A rather interesting finding by Tec was a very low percentage of marijuana users among students interested in athletics. He concludes from this that perhaps the undue emphasis placed on athletic achievement has merits beyond those usually recognized.

It is apparent that each adolescent must be individually evaluated as to the reasons for and the degree of his involvement in drug abuse. The blanket term of "drug abuser" by an agitated and bewildered nurse or physician adds nothing toward resolving this particular presenting complaint. Remember that 95 to 98 percent of young people who experiment with drugs do not get into any serious trouble. However, tragedies associated with drug abuse are not uncommon and each drug-abusing incident must be looked at as a potentially serious problem.

## THE NURSE'S ROLE IN DRUG ABUSE

Currently it is difficult for a nurse in a professional or private capacity to avoid the broad issue of drug abuse. Critical observation and appropriate intervention are vitally necessary for her in her dealings with drug abuse. Today, nurses find themselves dealing with drug-abuse issues in schools, public health facilities, "free medical clinics," drug maintenance and screening programs, emergency rooms, in-patient care, as well as in their private lives.

A 1970 survey by Lipp, Benson, and Allen demonstrated that a significant number of nursing students have used marijuana.[9] The direct danger to highly motivated young people in professional schools as a result of soft drug abuse is negligible. However, transposing such an attitude to the adolescent is obviously risky, as has been noted earlier. But at the same time, possessing a broad and relaxed perspective concerning drug abuse hopefully would enable one to be less likely to overreact to the problem, and instead to proceed with systematic evaluation and care.

## THE SCHOOL NURSE

The school nurse holds a prime position in relating to adolescents on a day-to-day basis. With the dramatic increase of drug abuse within the school system, the school nurse has had to incorporate a whole new set of ideas and behaviors into her school health activities. According to Caskey, Blaylock, and Wauson, defining her role in this area has not been an easy task.[10] For example, a school nurse who sees her role as primarily one of detecting and reporting drug abuse to the administration will behave differently from one who feels a deep responsibility for helping students find healthier ways to self-fulfillment. To function effectively, the role of the school nurse must be accepted by school administrators, teachers, and others on the health team.[10] For there is little evidence to support the hypothesis that drug-abuse education and prevention programs will significantly cause youth not to take the risk or expose themselves to the dangers of drug abuse.[11]

A school nurse who maintains the respect of the students and is known for her confidentiality and receptiveness will find herself a more effective teacher than any formal drug-abuse education program and will have little difficulty in times of crisis. Students will turn to her for help. As drug abuse is often a symptom of psychologic problems, an alert nurse within the school working closely with the teachers may be of aid in seeking early appropriate referral for the student. It should be noted that the normal mood swings of adolescents may be falsely attributed to drug abuse. Overreacting and labeling may be as psychologically devastating to the adolescent as not recognizing a serious drug reaction or overdose can be organically damaging.

Often a nurse, in addition to helping the staff decide the relative usefulness of educational approaches, correcting the defects in techniques used, and assisting in preparing an effective program, especially for the younger adolescent, can be particularly helpful to the individual youngster. The relaxed atmosphere of the nurse's office may be an acceptable neutral ground to discuss the issues of drug abuse. A school nurse who speaks with authority, but is not authoritarian, is a welcome addition to any school health program which is attempting to deal with drug abuse.

Drug-abuse counseling over any prolonged period may be highly complex and may depend on the differential factors of age, background, family, personality, situational variants, and individual reactions to the kinds of drugs abused. Nurses with adequate background and consultative support should become involved with prolonged counseling. However, genuine interest and availability during times of crisis may also be a highly effective means of dealing with short-term drug-abuse problems. Having developed an initially good rapport with a student, the nurse may help the adolescent to accept aid from other members of the health care team, especially in the area of psychotherapy.

Ordinarily students must be aware of, and give consent to, any notification of parents. If, however, concern over potential suicide or serious drug usage is present, a decision may have to be made to notify parents immediately. When the family does become involved, parents may need help in understanding the nature of the problem. Initial denial and anger may interfere with reaching a rational decision; family conflicts may often contribute to serious adolescent drug abuse. Adequate early referral of the student and his family may be facilitated by an effective school nurse.

The school nurse, as a primary member of the health care team, is in a vital position in which she can pick out the experimental, social, and occasional drug abuser. As mentioned previously, she is also well qualified to detect those young people who have psychologic problems and have turned to drugs either as a way of escaping from a life situation which has become intolerable or as a way of seeking a solution to their problems.

## TREATMENT AND REHABILITATION

Public attitude has changed concerning the treatment and rehabilitation of the drug abuser. This change has occurred in conjunction with the socioeconomic shift of drug abuse. Many American middle-class families have had a personal experience with this problem where formerly it was primarily associated with minority cultural groups of low economic stature. More emphasis is now being placed on treatment and rehabilitation than on the former punitive approach.

The virtual epidemic of drug abuse in the 1960s challenged the more traditional means of health care delivery. Many youthful drug abusers became alienated to the authoritarian defensive attitude of the medical profession. Emergency rooms were not equipped to "talk down" a hallucinating patient with his often equally incomprehensible peers.

The free clinic movement was begun by David E. Smith at the Haight-Ashbury psychedelic mecca in San Francisco in 1967.[12] One of its primary goals was to deliver acceptable health care to alienated youth. This system of predominantly volunteer support has now been established nationwide. The entree has become ready availability of medical care and the therapeutic milieu has turned into the "rap" session. Nurses, volunteer or salaried, have played a vital role in the free clinic movement. Each community-based effort has had to design a program to meet the specific needs of the area population. However, in a variety of settings, nurses have proven themselves to be highly able in caring for the youth in crisis, follow-up counseling, pregnancy detection and counseling, and assisting the physician in the diagnosis and treatment of venereal disease. The informal settings of such clinics have often led to the close association of all the members of a health care team.

The ability of the nurse to differentiate drug abuse from serious mental illness requires special expertise. Once acquired, the nurse may also play an important role in educating the medical community as well. Often mental health counselors are apt to be more effective if they work within a free clinic setting. "Rapping" is often alien to the classically trained social worker, psychologist, or other health care worker. Nurse clinicians may be of help to other health professionals in the use of rapping as a therapeutic technique.

An experienced full-time nurse offering continuity of care can be a stabilizing factor in a clinic in which volunteer physicians work. Although medical care may be delivered in a somewhat unorthodox manner, it is readily accepted by patients who use the clinic. Acceptance of mental health support is often a secondary but vital factor in treating clinic patients.

As a member of a health care team the nurse must be aware of other community resources. Often her youthful patients are runaways who demonstrate poor nutrition and are without food or shelter. Once confidence has been developed it is possible to refer the runaway to a shelter where parental reconciliation may occur.

## EMERGENCY CARE

Dr. Alfred Koumans, a staff psychiatrist at M.I.T. in Cambridge, Massachusetts, has stated that the medical profession has long been able to care for acute drug intoxication.[13] The difficulty with the current drug-abuse scene is not medical but instead, according to Dr. Koumans, social. As a result the extension of adequate medical care involves an increase in tolerance and a nonjudgmental approach to the drug culture. At the same time, however, this culture is constantly changing, as are the types of drugs being used. According to Foreman and Zerwekh, assessment is most effective when the patient and his friends accept the nurse as a concerned and understanding person.[14] The three major facets of assessment are contextual, behavioral, and physical.

The contextual setting can be established by finding out from the patient or his friends what particular drug he has taken. In addition, what has happened to the patient since the drug was taken is also important to know. Having teenagers milling about in an otherwise organized emergency room may challenge the nurse's organizing skill and patience to the utmost.

Behavioral observation should reflect the patient's moment-to-moment awareness, and any distortions in his mood and thought patterns as well as motor function.

As with any patient displaying alteration in consciousness or unstable vital signs, physical assessment involves careful and continuous monitoring of consciousness, pulse, respirations, temperature, blood pressure, pupil size, muscle tension, and gastrointestinal complaints. One must not lose sight of the possibility of CNS bleeding, infection, or metabolic disorders, all of which may complicate the symptoms of drug abuse or appear in their primary form.[14] Often the most alienated of adolescents are receptive to follow-up social and psychologic help if their crisis situations are handled well. Due to limited space the reader is referred for additional information to Koumans' Manual for the Treatment of Acute Drug Intoxication.[13]

A multitude of treatment programs have been developed in this country during the past ten years. The Public Health Service clinics in Fort Worth and Lexington have been ineffective as a result of their basic philosophy, which is the separation of the addict from his drug and community for a period of time.

Gay, Smith, and Shepard have described three major types of opiate-dependent individuals.[15] The first is the old-style junkie who is invariably black or a member of some other minority group with a socioeconomically deprived background. The individuals have a long history of repeated withdrawals and returns to narcotics. The second group consists of white middle-class addicts who started on nonaddicting agents but gradually gravitated to the use of heroin. The third group is termed the new junkie who experiments with and uses a wide variety of drugs.

Detection of these adolescents who are narcotic dependent is often difficult. As noted earlier, they are often the ones who drop out of school to support their habits.[5] Any nurse working with youth should maintain a high index of suspicion. Cutaneous manifestations of heroin addiction are often apparent. Serum hepatitis, withdrawal symptoms in the newborn infant of an unwed mother, arrests for prostitution or shoplifting may all point toward an individual involved in and supporting a narcotic habit.

Exploration of the pros and cons of methadone maintenance versus detoxification or involvement in a long-term therapeutic community is beyond the confines of this chapter. Rosenberg and Patch have noted the difficulty in treating adolescent heroin addicts.[16] They feel that the great majority do not achieve abstinence but become even more heavily involved with drugs and crime. Their experience with methadone maintenance among adolescents is that such treatment appeared to halt and even reverse the socioeconomic decay associated with long-term heroin use. This issue remains unresolved at this time.

The primarily nonadolescent methadone maintenance centers rely heavily on nursing care. Daily distribution of methadone is handled by the clinic nurse as is screening for the variety of physical and emotional symptoms that addicts display. The importance and responsibility of the nurse's role in a narcotic detoxification center are equally important.

## THE HOSPITALIZED ADDICT

Any patient admitted to a hospital unit could conceivably be drug dependent or, as he or she is more commonly called, a drug addict. Some addicts will probably not enter the hospital because of their drug problems but, rather, with a variety of medical conditions such as fractures, pregnancy, or any other medical or surgical problem that brings people to the hospital. Some, too, may be admitted because of complications from drug abuse, and with such conditions as hepatitis and various infections. And usually the drug addict who is hospitalized with a medical problem does not want "help" with his drug problem.

When a drug user is admitted for another medical problem, we must address ourselves to the treatment of this other problem. But the fact that the patient is a drug user poses an attitudinal difficulty among the health professionals involved in his care. And in fact, if we address ourselves too strongly to the drug problem, we are likely to "turn off" the patient and he will be less likely to continue to seek medical help for his other physical ailments. Thus each staff member must evaluate his or her own feelings and attitudes about this drug addicted patient and learn to deal with these feelings and attitudes appropriately. One way in which staff can be helped with these problems is through staff conferences.

Usually the hospitalized patient who is a drug user is very open in identifying himself as such to the physician taking the admission history. Since his illness may require extended hospitalization, the patient may need some kind of drug maintenance while in the hospital. Some health care professionals fear the drug addict and anticipate negative behavior. Actually the hospitalized addict is usually docile but manipulative with the staff as he tries to fulfill his desires and obtain his drug supply while in the hospital.

As has been noted throughout this chapter, the nurse who is involved with youth must be as aware of drug abuse as the nurse who is involved with drug abuse must be aware of the behavior of youth. To isolate one of these issues will be at the expense of the other and will often interfere with the primary goal. This relationship between drug abuse and youth is no easy problem and will be with us for many years ahead.

REFERENCES

1. Johnson KG, et al: Survey of adolescent drug use 1—Sex and grade distribution, AJPH 61:2418—32, 1971
2. Bogg RA, Smith RG, Russell SD: Drugs and Michigan High School students. Lansing, Michigan, Michigan Department of Public Health, 1969
3. Coddington RD, Jacobsen R: Drug use by Ohio adolescents. Ohio State Med J pp 481—84, 1972
4. Gossett JT, Lewis JM, Phillips VA: Extent and prevalence of illicit drug use as reported by 56,745 students. JAMA 216:1464—70, 1971
5. Porter MR, Vieira TA, Kaplan GJ, et al: Drug use in Anchorage, Alaska. JAMA 223:657—664, 1973
6. American Academy of Pediatrics, Committee on Youth: Drug Abuse in Adolescence, Pediatrics 44:131—41, 1969
7. Fine LL: What's a Normal Adolescent. Clin Pediatr (Phila) 12:1—5, 1973
8. Tec N: Some aspects of high school status and differential involvement with marihuana: A study of suburban teenagers. Adolescence 7:1—28, 1972
9. Lipp MR, Benson SG, Allen PS: Marihuana use by nurses and nursing students. Am J Nurs 71:2339—41, 1971
10. Caskey KK, Blaylock EV, Wauson BM: The school nurse and drug abusers. Nursing Outlook (New York) 18:27—30, 1970
11. Bourne PG: Is drug abuse a fading fad? J Am Coll Health Assoc 21:198—200, 1973
12. Smith DE, Rose AJ: Observations in the Haight-Ashbury medical clinic of San Francisco. Clin Pediatr (Phila) 7:313—16, 1968
13. Koumans AJR: Treatment of Acute Toxic Reactions to Abused Drugs. In Zarafonetis CJD (ed): Drug Abuse Proceedings of the International Conference. Philadelphia: Lea & Febiger, 1972, pp 381—84
14. Foreman NJ, Zerwekh JV: Drug crisis intervention, Am J Nurs 71:1736—41, 1971
15. Gay GR, Wellisch DK, Wesson R, et al: The psychotic junkie. Medical Insight pp 17—21, 1972
16. Rosenberg CM, Patch VD: Methadone use in adolescent heroin addicts. JAMA 220:991—93, 1972

# 8

# Approaches
# to Hospitalized Teenagers

AUDREY J. KALAFATICH AND ROBERT W. HERSHBERGER

There are many problems of, and with, hospitalized teenagers that are common to both boys and girls. However, the editor felt that there were enough differences to warrant two separate case presentations.

The first section is primarily concerned with a teenage girl who was undergoing treatment for scoliosis, a lateral curvature of the spine. The second section is concerned with male adolescents, and the case presented is a teenage boy who became a paraplegic following an auto accident. The nurse-author for the second section is a male nurse who participated in the nursing care of the patient discussed.

## GINNY: A THIRTEEN-YEAR-OLD IN A BODY CAST

By Audrey J. Kalafatich

The adolescent girl faces certain developmental tasks that she is expected to be dealing with during the adolescent period.

These include the acquisition of a sense of identity and the achievement of a degree of independence in preparation for assuming an adult role (these tasks are dealt with in more detail in Chapter 1). In addition to developmental tasks, any person who is sick has certain tasks to deal with. Nursing, as I see it, involves helping the individual to use whatever abilities she has to cope with whatever stresses face her as a result of her illness. And, hopefully, coping with these stresses can be a growth experience. This section attempts to answer the question "What does it mean to be a teenage girl and to be sick and hospitalized?" And, specifically, "How did one teenage girl and her mother cope with the problem of maintaining feminine identity while the girl was in a body cast?" During my work with hospitalized teenagers I became aware of the discrepancy between what they required for their development and what was demanded by their illness and/or treatment regime. I observed teenage girls whose bodies were almost completely encased in plaster casts during treatment for scoliosis. The cast extended down one leg to the knee. The head piece extension, used to immobilize the head, encircled it, with openings for the face and ears and the top of the head. The girls spent six weeks in the hospital undergoing the initial treatment which involved correction of the spinal curvature by means of the cast, called a Risser turnbuckle jacket, and surgery for spinal fusion. They faced the prospect of approximately ten months at home in bed in the cast in a recumbent position. Six of these months were to be spent in the Risser jacket and four more in a smaller body cast.

As stated previously, knowledge of adolescent psychosocial characteristics indicated an obvious discrepancy, and thus potential conflict, between behaviors which are characteristic of adolescence and the demands of the treatment. The first and most obvious treatment demand that conflicted with a normal adolescent characteristic was immobilization. Their large casts permitted the girls only gross movement from side to side. Adolescents are typically very physically active. One method frequently used by them to handle difficult situations is to take flight or withdraw. The adolescent, if possible, simply physically removes herself from the difficult situation. One 14-year-old girl, following application of her body cast, said to me, "I don't know what I'm going to do. Before, when my mother and I didn't get along, I'd simply leave. Now I won't be able to get away. I just don't know what I'm going to do!" During the time that the adolescent was in the cast undergoing treatment for scoliosis, not only was she immobilized and in a physically difficult situation but she also was denied one method, namely bodily activity, which she normally used to cope with such situations.

Second, as a result of its immobilizing quality the cast forced the adolescent to be almost totally dependent on others for such basic care as bathing. This enforced dependency created a situation for her that seems more typical for a much younger child. In fact, her need to be bathed while in the cast, and at times to be fed, resembled the dependency behaviors of an infant. This enforced dependency was occurring at a crucial time when the individual was struggling to be free from any dependency on family and other adults. The adolescent period is described as a time when it is necessary developmentally for the youth to try for ever increasing amounts of independence. Obviously, the treatment demands, in forcing a state of dependency, ran counter to the requisites of normal development.

Third, a treatment factor that appeared incongruous was that of the very purpose of the treatment. The treatment regime was directed at altering the body structure; more specifically, toward straightening the patient's back. Although the physician based the need for treatment on physiologic factors, the girls themselves verbalized cosmetic reasons for wanting the treatment. They submitted to the treatment because they wanted a "straight back." This reason given by the girls for undergoing the treatment obviously leads one to believe that they had already been self-conscious of their bodies and their deformities. The treatment was directed at artificially altering the body structure. Further, this superficial change in body structure was to be effectuated at a time when the individual was already struggling to incorporate the bodily changes normally occurring at adolescence into her body-image. These girls may or may not have already incorporated a crooked back into their body-images. Thus, in addition to the normal task of adolescence, that of adjusting to a normally changing body, the girls were subjected to surgical intervention which altered their present body structures.

Koegler[1] suggests "that corrective surgical procedures be performed before adolescence when this is feasible." But, medically, the ideal time for the correction of scoliosis is during early adolescence.[2] Spinal fusion, the surgical correction, is considered best done when the patient is approaching the completion of maximum growth and before her bony structure has become stabilized.

A fourth problem area with any hospitalized adolescent is that of the peer group. The peer group serves many functions. It offers support and also serves as a testing ground for the individual.[3] The peer group helps its members to cope with their changing bodies by offering a comparison group. In the same way, peer group members are helped with their strivings for independence. Each member of the group is able to compare her relationships with her parents and other adults with the way other members of the group handle similar relationships. Josselyn states " . . . in the peer group (the adolescent) can . . . find solace in the identical sufferings of others."[4] But, when the adolescent is hospitalized, she is deprived of the constant support of her regular peer group.

That the adolescent's dependency on the peer group is also manifested during hospitalization is documented in the literature.[5-7] Scofield[5(p 2)] found that peer groups were formed by adolescents in the hospital and that they serve the same purposes as for normal teenagers. But she confirmed problems of peer group formation due to the lack of availability of age-peers and the loss of friends as a result of discharges. On the other hand, Schechter[6] reported that strong friendships with peers developed in the hospital, and, in fact, he judged these to be stronger than those developed at home.

In summary, when the adolescent is hospitalized, there may be discrepancies between the developmental tasks and behaviors appropriate for that age and the demands imposed by the treatment regime. It therefore becomes imperative for the nurse working with hospitalized adolescents to be aware of normal adolescent tasks and behaviors and the discrepancies imposed by the treatment demands.

To illustrate several of the points made earlier in this section and to discuss the approaches used to deal with some of the problems of a hospitalized adolescent girl, I shall now offer some case material.* I would like to address the question: how did one 13-year-old girl named Ginny and her mother handle the developmental task of acquiring and maintaining for herself a body-image and also maintaining positive feelings about herself and her body-image when she was immobilized in a body cast for corrective scoliosis?

I first met Ginny V. on the day she was admitted to Children's Hospital in Pittsburgh for correction of her scoliosis. She was thirteen years old, had a fifteen-year-old brother, and lived with both parents. Her mother is an artist. Ginny's spinal curve was first noticed at seven years of age and progressed minimally until about six months prior to admission. Her pediatrician first noticed the defect when he "ran his finger down her spine." As Mrs. V. was reporting this information to me, Ginny interrupted her mother to say: "I

*Permission has been graciously granted by Ginny to allow me to share the data and the photographs of her.*

never could notice it!" Mrs. V. said that Ginny's father had the "same condition" and the resident physician reported later that he was told the father's condition was "unsuccessfully corrected." Also, Mrs. V. said that Ginny's fifteen-year-old brother had the condition but that it had not progressed. Ginny interrupted her mother to comment: "If I was a girl like him (referring to the severity of his deformity), I'd want to be corrected!" Mrs. V. commented on how much more concern there is over the physical appearance of girls.

Ginny had many adjustment problems with the cast itself as a result of its weight and mobility restrictions. After the initial adjustment period, however, both Ginny and her mother became primarily concerned with what Ginny "looked like" in the cast. Both continued to ponder how to maintain Ginny's femininity while she was in the body cast.

To give the reader some idea of the discrepancy, we present Figure 1 in which Ginny is seen prior to her hospitalization. She presents herself as a lovely, well-dressed young lady. Note that she is sitting in a position such that her uneven shoulders resulting from the deformity do not show. Also her dress has no waistline, hiding the fact that one of her hips is higher than the other.

In Figure 2, a cast similar to that used for Ginny's initial treatment is seen. The author is unaware whether the individual in the cast is a boy or a girl, and this answer cannot be determined from the photo. The lovely young lady in Figure 1 was faced with a monstrous cast like this. How can she *look* like a girl with *that* on?

The major problem therefore, was "How to help Ginny to look like a girl while she has to live in a large body cast?" Mrs. V. and I tried various methods, such as a poncho type outfit, which only managed to get bunched up as Ginny rolled around the bed. We also tried men's pajamas, as these were the only kind large enough to fit over the cast. But as Ginny so aptly put it, "How can one *look* like a *girl* in size 52 *men's* pajamas?"

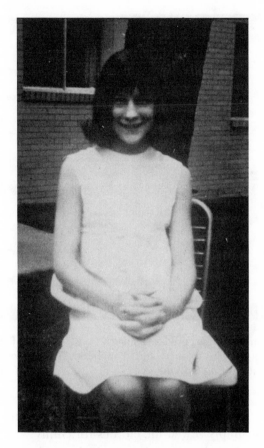

FIG. 1. Ginny prior to her hospitalization.

Ginny was discharged from the hospital with the primary problem being, as far as she was concerned, how to maintain her feminity while in a body cast.

Many phone calls were exchanged between Ginny's mother and myself with the recurring theme being questions regarding something for Ginny to wear *over* the cast. Remembering Mrs. V.'s artistic ability and creativity, I simply encouraged her by freely discussing with her the acknowledged need, and by reflecting "What do you think can be done?" Mrs. V.'s creativity resulted in what we referred to as

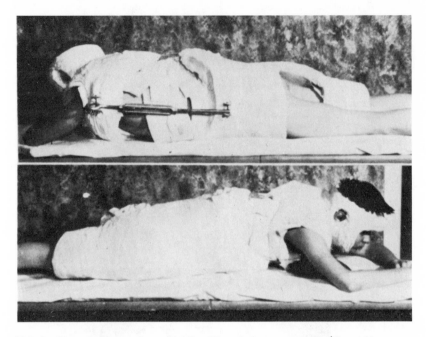

FIG. 2. Cast similar to that used for Ginny's first treatment (From Ferguson: Orthopedic Surgery in Infancy and Childhood, 1963. Courtesy of The Williams and Wilkins Co., Publishers.)

Ginny's "outfits." She had made a pattern using newspaper, and then simply sewed the clothes for Ginny.

In Figure 3, Ginny is seen in her "picnic outfit." This was initially appropriate because she was put into the cast in July.

In September, Ginny had a tutor come to her home so that she could keep up with her school work. This necessitated her "school outfit" as seen in Figure 4.

In October I received a phone call from Mrs. V. and she expressed concern about a Halloween celebration. I again simply offered encouragement. Ginny had a Halloween party in her home and everyone invited came in costume, and Ginny was in costume too. A sheet was draped over her cast and a hair piece provided long hair. A bowl of grapes completed the "Cleopatra floating down the Nile outfit"!

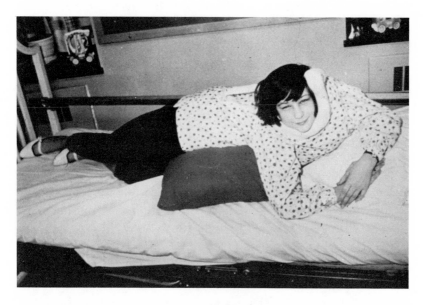

FIG. 3. Ginny in her "picnic outfit."

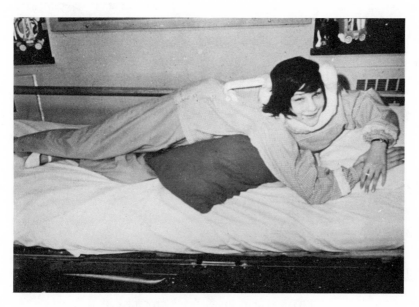

FIG. 4. Ginny in her "school outfit."

The holiday season brought the need for a "party outfit." Figure 5 shows Ginny in her "pink brocade." She really looked lovely and my comment was that all she needed to be dressed for any fancy ball was to have a string of pearls around her neck! Her response was "Do you think we could find one long enough?"

I would like the reader to note that in Figures 3, 4, and 5 Ginny is wearing shoes. She was not permitted to stand and in fact remained in the horizontal position the entire time she was in the cast. But remember, these outfits were an attempt to help Ginny to retain as much as possible the features of a "normal girl." I asked Ginny about the shoes and her reply was, "Don't you wear shoes?" Thus Ginny, upon awakening in the morning, got completely dressed just like any other "normal girl."

After six months in the cast, Ginny returned to the hospital and a smaller walking cast was applied, extending from the axilla to the hips. Figure 6 shows Ginny upon

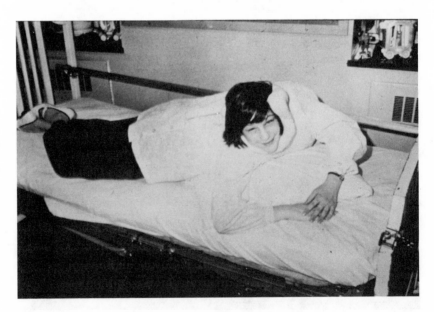

FIG. 5. Ginny in her "pink brocade."

discharge following this second hospitalization. She is wearing an orange-colored shift with an orange ribbon in her hair, still looking very feminine.

Figure 7 shows Ginny two years later. Note the difference in her posture from that shown in Figure 1. In this photograph her straight back is displayed, the attainment of the primary goal in her treatment regime.

Not all who enter the system for health care live "happily ever after." But this family's ability to cope made a stressful treatment regime only one incident in a youngster's life and made it possible for her to move on in her overall development.

This case study would not be complete without a comment on where Ginny is now. In correspondence with her about this chapter, I asked for a recent photo. She sent

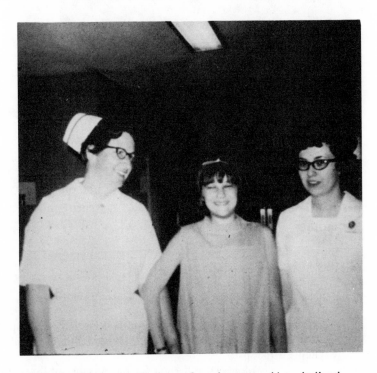

FIG. 6. Ginny upon discharge from her second hospitalization.

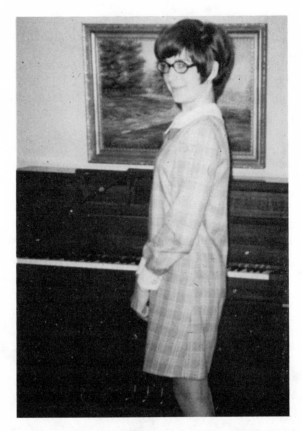

FIG. 7. Ginny two years after her hospitalization.

the one shown in Figure 8, which shows her on her way to her high school senior prom, and she is wearing another of her mother's "creations."

REFERENCES

1.  Koegler R: Chronic illness and the adolescent. Ment Hyg 44, New York, 1960, p 114
2.  Donaldson WF Jr: Scoliosis. In Ferguson R Jr (ed): Orthopedic Surgery of Infancy and Childhood, 2nd ed. Baltimore, Williams & Wilkins, 1963, p 197
3.  Committee on Adolescence, Group for the Advance of Psychiatry:

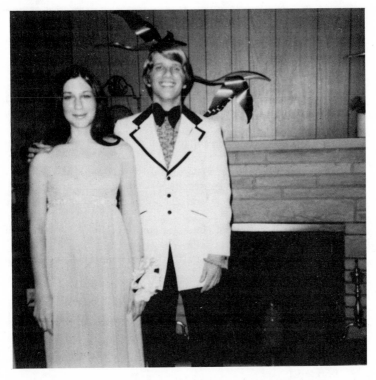

FIG. 8. Ginny on her way to her high school senior prom.

Normal Adolescence: Its Dynamics and Impact. New York, Scribner's, 1968
4. Josselyn I: The Adolescent and His World. New York, Family Service Association of America, 1952
5. Scofield C: Adolescents in the hospital. Maternal Child Nursing Conference, University of Pittsburgh, School of Nursing, June 1966, p 1
6. Schechter M: The orthopedically handicapped child; emotional reactions. Arch Gen Psych Vol IV, Mar 1961, p 250
7. Bergman T: Children in the Hospital. New York, International U Press, 1965

BIBLIOGRAPHY

Abend S et al: Reactions of adolescents to short-term hospitalization. Am J Psychiatry 124:7, Jan 1968, pp 109–14

Bergman T: Children in the Hospital. New York, International U Press, 1965

Blake F: Immobilized youth: a rationale for supportive nursing intervention. Am J Nurs 69:11, Nov 1969, pp 2364–69

Byers ML: The hospitalized adolescent. Nurs Outlook 17:8, Aug 1969, pp 32–34

Committee on Adolescence, Group for the Advancement of Psychiatry: Normal Adolescence: Its Dynamics and Impact. New York, Scribner's, 1968

Conway B: The effects of hospitalization on adolescence. Adolescence, Vol 6, 1971, pp 77–92

Duran MT: Family-centered care and the adolescent's quest for self-identity. Nurs Clin North Am, 7:1, Mar 1972, pp 65–73

Koegler RR: Chronic illness and the adolescent. Ment Hyg, Vol 44, Jan 1960, pp 111–14

Mason EA: The hospitalized child—his emotional needs. N Eng J Med, Vol 272, Feb 25, 1965, pp 406–14

Myers BA, Friedman SB, Weiner IB: Coping with a chronic disability. Am J Dis Child 120:3, Sept 1970, pp 175–81

Schonfeld WA: Body-image in adolescents: a psychiatric concept for the pediatrician. Pediatrics, Vol 31, May 1963, pp 845–55

Schowalter JE, Lord RD: The hospitalized adolescent. Children 18:4, July–Aug 1971, pp 127–32

Scofield C: Adolescents in the hospital. Maternal Child Nursing Conference, University of Pittsburgh, School of Nursing, June 1966, pp 1–4

## NICK: A SIXTEEN-YEAR-OLD NEW PARAPLEGIC

By Robert W. Hershberger

Unlike the child with a birth defect or progressive disabling disease, the adolescent who experiences disability as a result of injury must cope with sudden loss of body function. He has no time to prepare for hospitalization, and separation from family and peers. The adolescent's life style and plans must be modified. The degree of modification depends upon the severity of the disability as well as the adolescent's emotional response. For the adolescent already struggling to construct a new body-image, to establish independence and sexual identity, and to prepare for adult social and vocational roles, a sudden physical disability drastically increases the difficulty of his task.

Adolescence is a period during which the self-concept, in which body-image plays a prominent role, undergoes change. According to Schonfeld,[1] normal adolescence requires radical reconstruction of body-image because of rapid changes in size, body proportions, and primary and secondary sexual characteristics occurring with pubescence.

The adolescent's intensified awareness of his body is attributed to consciousness of his own physical development, to inflated emphasis assigned to physical traits by peers, and to increasing identification with culturally determined standards. The adolescent is extremely sensitive about his concept of self and reacts with instant responsiveness to what he thinks of himself and to what others think of him. Since his image of self is in a state of flux, approval or disapproval by others assumes a critical importance.[1]

Consequently the adolescent who experiences disability as a result of injury is faced with a severe psychologic loss which tends to undermine his self-esteem and drastically change his body-image. Gunther contends that the individual's body-image may be one of the earliest fundamental components of the human ego and that, as a result of physical mutilation or injury, the ego is only very slowly able to alter its concept of what the changed body looks like.[2] Likewise, when the status value of body-whole, body-well, and body-beautiful is high, a physical disability may be so traumatic to the individual that he is completely unable to integrate his new physique into his self-concept.[3]

Adolescence can be considered an overlapping situation, consisting of both child and adult components of accepted behavior. The concept of overlap also is useful to describe the psychologic world of the handicapped. This individual is subject to the mores and expectations of the disabled group, but his wish is to be just like anyone else. When these two determinants of behavior are incompatible, then inconsistent, emotional, and exaggerated behavior can be expected.[3(pp 156-67)]

The adolescent with a disability, then, must cope with two types of persistent overlap situations: one owing to his disability and one owing to his transitional status as a child-adult. The disability itself may tend to prolong the period of adolescence by delaying the emotional separation from parents. In our society the status of full adulthood generally is withheld until the individual can assume economic independence and the responsibilities of marriage.[3(pp 185-86)]

The developmental task concept of Havighurst is useful when considering the effects of illness or disability on an adolescent. Havighurst views both living and growing as learning processes. Developmental tasks take on the nature of both individual need and social demand in that they arise from the combination of physical maturation, cultural pressures, and the desires, goals, and values of the individual. Havighurst lists the developmental tasks of adolescence, the period from twelve to eighteen years of age, as follows:

1. Achieving new and more mature relations with age mates of both sexes
2. Achieving a masculine or feminine social role
3. Accepting one's physique and using one's body effectively
4. Achieving emotional independence from parents and other adults
5. Achieving assurance of economic independence

6. Selecting an occupation and preparing for it
7. Preparing for marriage and family life
8. Developing intellectual skills and concepts necessary for civic competence
9. Desiring and achieving socially responsible behavior
10. Acquiring a set of values and an ethical system as a guide to behavior[4]

The adolescent with a physical disability may have difficulty learning some of these developmental tasks.

The purpose of this section is to describe the behavior characteristics of a male adolescent hospitalized for paraplegia that was induced by the trauma of an automobile accident. The adolescent is Nick, a sixteen-and-one-half-year-old with whom I worked for the first twelve weeks after he had his accident. Some of Nick's behavior could be related to his disability.

Nick's injury occurred as a result of a hitchhiking adventure. On a Saturday afternoon in autumn, Nick and his friend Bill decided to take a hitchhiking trip. Nick and Bill were picked up by an adolescent in a new blue car. Later Nick fell asleep in the back seat of the car. His friend Bill drove since the other adolescent was tired of driving. The adolescent told Bill that he was only fourteen years old, that he did not have a driver's license, and that he had stolen the car. A couple of hours later, the three youths were pursued by the police because Bill had gone through a red light. The boys were frightened and tried to outrun the police. Nick later reported that he awoke just in time to realize that they were attempting to escape. They were traveling over ninety miles per hour when Bill lost control of the car and it crashed through a guard rail and flipped over several times. Bill was uninjured but Nick was thrown from the car and landed unconscious in the median strip. The adolescent who stole the car was also injured and was taken with Nick to a small local hospital in southern Ohio. Nick was given emergency treatment but plans were made to transfer him to a larger hospital due to the extent and nature of his injuries.

Nick was transferred to the University Hospitals in

Columbus. The diagnosis was established that he had bilateral hemopneumothorax, two ribs fractured posteriorly, fracture and dislocation of the fourth, fifth, and sixth thoracic vertebrae, and probably a severed spinal cord at the level of the fourth thoracic vertebra. Nick was admitted to the neurosurgical patient care unit. My contact with Nick and his family began later that morning.

During the course of Nick's hospitalization, I learned much about his family relationships and life style. He described his family as being "packed together and sarcastic about each other." The family consisted of Nick's father and stepmother, their two-and-one-half-year-old daughter, five adolescents from previous marriages, and an infant daughter of Nick's unmarried half-sister. Nick described his father as "the nicest man I know" and appeared to have a good relationship with his stepmother. Nick felt there was no "generation gap" in his family because his parents were realistic about the children's smoking, drinking, and sexual activity. Yet he felt that his parents did care about his activities. Unlike most adolescents, Nick never spoke disrespectfully or critically of his parents.

Nick's parents described Nick as being very independent and "a loner." They felt Nick did not make friends readily or confide in anyone; that he was "manipulative" and "could talk people into anything." Nick had been brought before the court for juvenile delinquency and had been on probation for awhile. He dropped out of school and became increasingly defiant and difficult for his parents to control. Nick sometimes prepared his own food rather than eat with the family. He made no attempt to find a job. He slept and lived in one set of clothes for weeks at a time and refused to get his hair cut. Yet his parents felt that "if we had to choose anyone of our kids to stand by us through thick or thin, it would be Nick." Some of Nick's behavior could be attributed to his desire not to be dependent on his family; however, he did not learn to develop his independence always in desirable ways. Throughout his hospitalization, Nick's family was very supportive and attentive. They visited him almost every weekend. They were concerned about Nick's physical and vocational rehabilitation and remained quite sensitive to his emotional needs.

## WEEK 1

I first saw Nick on Sunday morning, about twenty hours after his accident. Nick had been admitted to the neurosurgical patient care unit at the University Hospitals in Columbus and had been placed in a four-bed ward. He was lying on his back on a Stryker frame. He had rather long brown hair, a light but muscular physique, and was five feet, eight inches tall. He was receiving blood in one arm and intravenous fluids in the other. Both arms were restrained. He had skin abrasions on his head, neck, arms, and legs. A nasogastric tube, a Foley catheter, and bilateral chest tubes were in place. Nick was drowsy and kept his eyes closed most of the time. He responded to his name and sometimes to questions. At other times he was confused and irrational, pulling at his restraints and yelling, "I want to get out of here." He had sensation down to about two inches below the nipple line and was arcflexic and without motor function in the lower extremities. Bowel and bladder control were gone.

Nick's father and brother had spent the night at the hospital with him and expressed much concern about him. The physicians had told them that Nick's condition was critical, that probably his spinal cord was severed, and that a spinal fusion would be necessary to stabilize the fracture in Nick's spine. I answered their questions about Nick's nursing care and provided clarification, at times just listening as the two struggled with the impact of Nick's condition and prognosis.

I provided the physical nursing care for Nick on

Tuesday morning. Nick was lethargic and slept almost continuously unless stimulated. He seemed to wake up only when I would verbally try to make him respond. Range of motion for his extremities and a bowel training program were initiated. He began taking ice chips and sips of water. He hallucinated at times, but generally responded more rationally to questions. As the day progressed, he became more alert and oriented. Later his father and brother visited. Encouraged by Nick's improvement, they planned to go home that afternoon.

When I returned on Friday, Nick was alert and oriented. He did not remember me from my contact with him on Tuesday morning, but he did recall his father telling him about me before leaving for home Tuesday afternoon. Nick was eager to talk and did not even stop when his mail was delivered. He talked about his part-time jobs and activities during the summer. He described his home town, his home, and his family. Nick mentioned that he had witnessed his real mother being murdered four days before his twelfth birthday and that the murderer had been caught and sent to prison. He told the story unemotionally yet in a confiding manner. I was somewhat shocked by his story and the life style he described for himself. I interpreted his disclosure as an indication of trust in me. I listened attentively, tried to remain nonjudgmental in my reactions, and commented that the experience must have been very difficult for him.

Nick later talked about his hitchhiking trip and the accident. He had learned the details of the accident on Wednesday from the parents of the adolescent who had stolen the car. Nick said he "wasn't too clear about what was going on" until shortly before his father left Tuesday afternoon. His voice was hoarse, apparently as a result of irritation from the nasogastric tube which had already been inserted for two days. Nick felt that his voice was also affected by his lying in bed this long and commented, "I'm used to being on my feet all the time." I responded that being suddenly confined to bed did require an adjustment.

Nick had been placed on a liquid diet. He was able to be turned on the Stryker frame since Wednesday, when the left chest tube was removed. As a result of lying on his back continuously during the first four days after the accident, skin breakdown had occurred over his coccyx and the hunched portion of the vertebral column at the fracture site. Special skin care measures and frequent turning were instituted to treat and prevent further skin breakdown.

## WEEK 2

By the following Monday the intravenous infusion in Nick's right arm had been discontinued and he was placed on a selective diet. He had learned how to adjust the arm rest and table on the Stryker frame for his comfort and convenience. He began to assist with the positioning of pillows and tubes in preparation for turning. He was concerned about the effect of his hospitalization on his family's finances, and commented, "That helps a lot—me in the hospital right after Ma quit her job." He described what he could remember of his one previous hospitalization at four-and-one-half years of age. He commented that he thought removal of his Foley catheter would be as painful as was the removal of the intravenous catheter from his arm. He was eager for his physician to remove the right chest tube because "then they'll fix my back for me. Then I'll be able to sit up and look out that window." In accordance with the philosophy of patient care on this neurosurgical patient care unit, Nick was not told initially that he had suffered damage and probable severing of the spinal cord which would probably result in permanent paraplegia. Nick's questions about his injury were to be answered frankly and honestly when he asked for information or clarification. It was believed that this would allow him to reach his own conclusions at a pace with which he could cope.

On Tuesday morning, Nick was quiet, somber, and uncommunicative for a few hours. Several times when I left the room and returned, I found him with his eyes closed. He denied being tired. He referred to his back as being "injured" and acknowledged having "no feeling or movement" below the level of injury. He described the sensation of knowing the position of his feet and legs even though actual sensation was absent. He assisted with his bath, and combed his hair and shaved. Nick's right chest tube had been removed during the night. Chest X-rays following removal of the chest tube showed a 20 percent pneumothorax on the right. As a result, a thoracentesis was performed that evening which proved to be a frightening and painful experience for Nick. He later described the procedure as being "really rough and I don't want another one."

By Friday, Nick was again talkative and cheerful. The occupational therapist had visited him and planned with him to begin woodcraft activity. Nick was eager to see his family on the weekend and had obtained permission for his two-and-one-half-year-old sister to visit him. He had started to read a novel and to watch a roommate's television in the evenings. He talked about his experiences of working for a circus carnival during a past summer. He discussed some of his hitchhiking trips and commented, "Everyplace I go, I hitchhike. I love to hitchhike. (pause) I did." He appeared to have some doubt that he would be able to hitchhike in the future. Nick was also concerned that his hair had not been washed since his accident. I washed Nick's hair and planned with him to wash his hair every Tuesday morning thereafter. I viewed his interest in his physical appearance as a typical adolescent concern.

During this second week of hospitalization, Nick appeared to be interested in asserting his independence and learning about various aspects of his physical care. He struggled with the reality of his accident, his hospitalization, and separation from his family. He seemed unable to focus on the actual injury or to understand the significance of the loss of function and sensation. Yet Nick did appear to be giving some thought to the meaning of his back injury when he implied that hitchhiking might not be possible in the future.

Nick gave the impression of being at times a worldly, confident young man, yet at other times of being a frightened, threatened child. His behavior is characteristic of an adolescent's struggle between wanting to be independent and wanting to be dependent. This illustrates how adolescence can be considered an overlap situation, as the individual has both an adult and a child component of acceptable behavior.[3](pp 156-67)

## WEEK 3

During the weekend, the neurosurgeon had informed Nick and his family that the spinal fusion could probably be performed in about a week since Nick's respiratory complications were responding to treatment. Nick was able to be transported on the Stryker frame to the physical therapy and occupational therapy departments. I felt that being transported to other departments was important because it represented to Nick an increased mobility and was also a definite change of environment. Nick continued to assist with his physical care and began to remind nursing personnel of the scheduled times for turning. I assisted nursing personnel on the unit to recognize this behavior as a means for Nick to maintain independence. Nick wanted to get a new twelve-string guitar which he could use in the hospital since his other guitar was electric and required the use of an amplifier. He hoped to borrow the money for the guitar from his older sister and commented, "I'll be able to pay her back in about ten months with my job and everything." Regarding his part-time job as a busboy which he had obtained two weeks before the accident, he commented, "I plan on keeping that. That's a nice job." He talked about his plan to go to California this past summer, his parents' resultant petition to the court to prevent him from going, and his eventual decision to return to his home town high school. He said, "Yeah, I'm going back [to school] this year in January."

Nick was interested in and concerned about his three roommates. Particularly the one roommate who had a brain tumor. Nick heard the neurosurgeons explain that this man might become paralyzed as a result of having surgery to remove the tumor. Nick remarked, "He's got more guts than I do because I'd rather live with a tumor than be paralyzed. (pause) Then again, I've got to face surgery myself." He hesitated again, then changed the subject.

While giving care to Nick on Tuesday morning I explained that after his spinal fusion he would eventually be able to get up in a wheelchair and would then be able to handle more of his own care. And that he could continue with some of his current interests, such as playing the guitar. No discussion occurred as to whether or not use of the wheelchair would be permanent. Nick commented, "You have to sit somewhere when you play the guitar, so the wheelchair should work out OK." He had begun writing letters to his family and friends. When I asked what he had written about his injury, he replied, "Not too much. Just that I broke my back, but that I'm OK."

Nick commented, "It won't be long before I can get out of bed and then I'll be using my arms more than my legs. So I have to build up the muscles." I explained to him that he would be getting out of bed, but that this would occur after healing following the spinal fusion. Nick was quiet for a moment, then said slowly and hesitantly, "Well . . . I think what it is . . . well . . . my back is busted. It's pinching my spine. That's why I don't have any feeling. My feeling stops right where my back is busted. . . . So, I think after they fix my back, I'll have feeling . . . throughout my body." I asked if Nick could be sure that the surgery would give him his feeling back. Nick replied,

I'm not positive . . . that I'll ever . . . have feeling back. The way I figure it, it's just that it's pinching my spine . . . and that's what's making me numb. I have high hopes that that's what it is. And when they fix my back, it will automatically put the feeling back . . . 'cause it'll take the pressure off my spine. I'm just hoping that's what's wrong and that's how it works out.

I was excited that Nick had reached this increased awareness of his injury. I also suddenly felt frightened and inadequate in helping him to cope with his realizations. I responded that his conclusions could possibly be correct. Because of my anxiety about dealing with Nick's awareness of his paralysis, I asked him what specific fears he had about surgery. Nick replied,

For one thing, all the needles involved. After that is the fact that they are messing with my spine . . . Just one little slip could really mess me up for life . . . if I'm not messed up already . . . and I don't think I am . . . already.

I commented that Nick seemed to be aware that his spinal cord might already be damaged. Nick said,

I recognized that [spinal cord involvement] as soon as I realized where I was and why I was there. I recognized that there could be a lot of damage already done. When I first woke up, I started testing to find out where I had feeling . . . and where I didn't. The first thing I thought of was my eyesight . . . because I realize how important eyesight is. That was the first thing I checked. Then I checked my hands because of my guitar. If I didn't have music, I think I'd die. So I checked my hands and arms, and then I tried to move my legs and they wouldn't move. So I started to feel and noticed I couldn't feel either. So, then, I felt the pain in my back. And I figured right then . . . that something had happened to my spine.

When I commented that the possibility of not walking again must be very frightening, Nick replied, "Well, I'm kinda

keeping my mind negative. Ya know, I'm not . . . positive . . . either way, and I don't think about it . . . that much.
I try to keep it out of my mind . . . as much as possible." A
few tears rolled down his cheeks, but Nick continued,

> I learned when I was eleven years old when my mother got
> killed . . . that you have to face up to things . . . take 'em as they
> are . . . I realized it then, and I've more or less beat it into myself
> that when something happens, you've got to take it. There's no
> way to change it.

Nick told about witnessing his mother's being murdered
and described how he maintained control and hid his younger
brother and himself from the gunman. He felt that his past
experiences had made him strong "mentally" and I reinforced his conclusion.

The apparent inability to think about or understand the
finality of his injury probably protected Nick from acute
anxiety. When Nick commented that he would rather live
with a tumor than be paralyzed, he appeared to be trying to
understand the horror of the trauma that had occurred. He
began to refer to his back as being "broken" while earlier he
had referred to his back as being "injured," and he was able
to consider the necessity for using a wheelchair in the future.
Yet he seemed unable to understand the significance of his
broken back. Finally, almost three weeks after the injury,
Nick was able to discuss the conclusions he had reached
about his injury. During the second week he had hinted at
knowing that he might not walk again. Now he displayed
anxiety while discussing his broken back and the possibility
of spinal cord damage. He seemed to be acutely threatened
by the possibility of permanent disability and he tried not to
think about it. Nick seemed to be trying to convince himself
that he had dealt with harsh reality before (his mother's
murder) and therefore could face and accept his current
situation, though almost overwhelming.

## WEEK 4

In contrast to his anxiety last Friday, Nick was generally calm and relaxed on Monday and Tuesday of this week. He had finished reading a second novel and planned to have his family bring his record player and albums to the hospital. He was trying to respond to the many cards and letters he had received. He talked at length about his family's visit over the weekend.

Nick was interested in the rationale for a bowel training program and began to determine for himself when a suppository was needed. But he remarked, "I would rather go to the bathroom. If I get my feeling back, I'll be able to. I hope that I will." During range of motion exercises to his legs, he said, "They sure are thinner. I want to keep them built up so if I get my feeling back, I'll be able to walk." He added jokingly, "Maybe I'll have to hitchhike in a wheel-chair." He described a relative who was injured in Vietnam. The relative was paralyzed from the waist down, had lost bowel and bladder control, and was confined to a wheelchair, all of which Nick characterized as being "a terrible thing for that guy."

On Friday, Nick announced, "I think I'm getting my feeling back." He reported being able at times to feel the padding under his buttocks and the coolness of solutions applied to his coccyx. He began to irrigate his Foley catheter on his own and to keep a record of his oral fluid intake. He contemplated staying at the University Hospitals for his rehabilitation after surgery rather than being transferred to a physical rehabilitation facility nearer his home.

The neurosurgical resident physician came in to discuss the spinal fusion with Nick. He informed Nick that the surgery would occur in about ten days and he referred to Nick as being paralyzed. Nick became subdued and repeatedly pulled at the skin on his neck as he listened intently.

The resident physician remarked that Nick was probably already thinking that he may not get his feeling back. Nick replied that he had concluded that he had a "fifty-fifty chance" of getting his feeling back. The resident then explained that Nick's chance was not even that good and that, most likely, he would not get his feeling back and he would not be able to walk again.

After the resident left, Nick talked slowly and quietly, and a few tears ran down his cheeks. I felt rather powerless and very sad. He explained what he understood about the surgery.

> They're just gonna fuse my back together . . . and whether or not my feeling comes back . . . that's less than a fifty-fifty chance. It's not what I thought it was, but there's nothing they can do about that. So if it does come back, it'll just be a by-product of the operation. I'm glad they're honest instead of saying, "We're pretty sure it'll come back, and get my hopes up. Still, I'd rather have it [surgery] while I know . . . rather than have 'em build me up, then let me down . . . But still a wheelchair is better than a bed for the rest of my life. And like you said, I've got good hands. I can still play the guitar.

Nick then turned to a discussion of his relative who had paraplegia and explained, "He's paralyzed, well . . . just about the way I am from here (pointing to his lower chest) on down." He began to discuss how his life might be changed by the paralysis. "I know for one thing, if I don't get my feeling back, I won't be able to hitchhike, but I will be able to drive." He explained that his relative had hand controls on his car. "As long as I'm able to get one of those, I'll be able to drive. At least I can still travel, 'cause that's one of my main interests in life." After a long pause, he continued, "It won't be too easy to find the kind of job I like. I'll have to give up the job I have now . . . if I don't get my feeling back. Still, there are other jobs . . . If I can't find a job one place, I can always go someplace else and try it."

Nick then launched into a long discussion of his interest and possible career in music. He had written over fifty songs and felt that he could sell ten or fifteen of them. His guitar playing was self-taught and he did not read music. He had started playing the guitar three years ago. He commented, "That's one thing that I don't think will interfere . . . wheelchair or no wheelchair. I'll still be able to sit a guitar in my lap or else on the arm of the chair." Another problem Nick identified was that his bedroom at home was upstairs. He reported that he had worked hard to plan and arrange his bedroom and he did not want to give it up. He also indicated that a step between the dining room and kitchen would be a barrier to wheelchair mobility. He paused for a moment, then seemed reflective,

I'm just keeping my fingers crossed that I don't have to use the wheelchair for the rest of my life. I did realize that I might . . . and now I have to realize that I probably will [have to use the wheelchair] . . . There's quite a difference there. Still, if I do, I do.

Later Nick mentioned his fear of surgery and remarked, "I want to know what to expect." I planned with Nick to concentrate on preoperative teaching during the following week.

The data from this fourth week indicated that Nick was struggling to face the reality of his injury and resultant disability, but his endeavor continued to be hindered by an inability to understand or think logically about his situation. Early in the week his anxiety appeared low in contrast to the anxiety he manifested on the previous Friday. He tended to focus on his family's visit, the location for future rehabilitation, aspects of physical care, and other nonthreatening facets of the situation rather than on the meaning and implications of his injury. He could even joke about hitchhiking in a wheelchair. These appeared to be defensive maneuvers serving temporarily to lower anxiety. His use of the expression "if I get my feeling back" seemed to be a technique for acknowledging the possibility that he might be paralyzed. In his reference to "the terrible thing" that his paraplegic relative had experienced, Nick may have projected his own reaction from being in a similar situation.

Nick appeared to be experiencing denial when he said that he thought he was getting his feeling back. He had expressed sincere hope that sensation would return, and as a result of his wishful thinking, he imagined that sensation appeared to be returning. His expressed denial was almost concomitant with increased and progressive awareness. Nick concluded that he had only a "fifty-fifty chance" of getting his feeling back, when earlier he had considered it as a distinct possibility. When the neurosurgeon discussed the surgery with him, Nick was abruptly confronted with the fact of paralysis and the expectation that he would not walk again. He became very anxious afterward; he was "torn up" by that confrontation. He had been unable before logically to associate his loss of feeling and function with paralysis. Now he referred to himself as being paralyzed just like his relative. He was able to identify and discuss several problems which paralysis would present. He would be unable to hitchhike, and employment, driving, and his upstairs bedroom presented special difficulties. He appeared to be trying to understand how his life would be changed, but he could not think about this very long. The focus of his conversation alternated from future concerns to those less threatening or to past interests and events. Nick wanted to drive a car, keep his upstairs bedroom, and maintain a job—all typical concerns of the adolescent as he strives for independence. However, Nick could not discuss those concerns without changing topics or resorting to joking as a means of attempting to cope.

During the early part of the week Nick appeared to be much more composed and at ease than he had been on the preceding Friday. He finished a wall plaque in occupational therapy. He had been loaned a guitar to use for the duration of his hospitalization, and he played it with enthusiastic devotion. Although he had not smoked since his accident, he now took it up again. Nick began to experience muscle spasms in his legs and was interested in how and why they occurred. He discussed his fears related to surgery: the intravenous catheter insertion, waking up during surgery, and pain. He focused intermittently on the plans for his preoperative and postoperative care. I informed him of future rehabilitation concerns such as bowel and bladder care, transfer techniques, dressing, skin care, and vocational preparation.

Nick expressed concern for a young woman recently admitted to the unit following an automobile accident. He explained, "She broke her back like I did . . . She will probably end up with the same surprises I've ended up with. Maybe I could help her out a little bit—explain and give her a few hints on what's gonna happen to her." I commented that he might have opportunities to talk with her but cautioned that she would need time to reach her own conclusions about her injury as he had done. His altruistic intention was typical for an adolescent but was also probably used by Nick as a means of coping with his own injury.

By Friday the orthopedic surgeon had scheduled Nick's surgery for the following Monday and had discussed the surgery and postoperative plans with him. Nick reported that the surgeon had told him he would remain on the Stryker frame for six or seven weeks after surgery, at which time he would be fitted with a back brace, and could go home after learning to use the wheelchair. He commented,

> So now I'm not nearly as scared about surgery as I was before, but I'm still smoking more as it gets closer . . . I've got a lot of confidence in my doctors . . . Before I was scared half out of my mind and now it doesn't even bother me hardly.

He joked about missing breakfast and the "vampire" (laboratory technician) on the morning of surgery. He had decided that he would ask his parents to let him go to Dodd Hall, the physical rehabilitation facility of the medical center, for a few weeks of rehabilitation rather than transfer to a facility nearer his home. He explained again that he would be able to go home a few weeks after the point where he could get up in a wheelchair.

> After I get off the Stryker frame, I don't think it will take more than two or three weeks to learn to use the wheelchair. I'm a pretty quick learner when I want to be. The main thing I'm going to have to learn is to get around without my legs . . . I mean, that's if I don't get my legs . . . As soon as I learn to throw my body around without using my legs, then I'll be doing OK. So, it will only take me, I figure, a couple of weeks at the most—maybe three weeks—to learn to use the wheelchair.

When I explained that rehabilitation involved more than learning to use the wheelchair, Nick retorted,

> The main thing they're gonna have to help me do is to get out of a mud hole if I get stuck, (laugh) 'cause in the springtime it gets real muddy around home. And crippled or not crippled, I'm not gonna stay in the house. I love nature and even if I just have to sit out in the woods, I'm still gonna enjoy the beauty of the woods—and the beauty of winter—And I'm still gonna go swimming. Swimming and fishing I've got all figured out. I can swim one-quarter of a mile . . . I never use my feet when I swim—just my arms, 'cause all my strength is in my arms. That's one reason why I'm glad I've got them left . . . I love to swim and that's one thing I won't give up. Mom or Dad can take me down

to the lake and wade out to their waists and carry me into the water ... Fishing I already have a cure for, cause they have eight-foot aluminum boats ... So I'll just row around until I can get a three horse power motor ... The only thing I'm gonna need is transportation and somebody to carry me into the boat and pick me up when I'm through fishing.

Nick expounded on the strength of his arms and how he had outworked three other men stacking bales of hay and how he had carried one-hundred pound bags of grain with ease. Then he returned to analyzing his situation.

I've already figured out ways to do just about everything I want to do except hitchhiking. And I'll never be able to hitchhike again if I don't get my legs back ... And I'm still praying and hoping that I get my legs back ... yet I know what my chances are, but I'm still hoping. Just because I found out that my chances are slimmer than what I thought, doesn't mean that I can't keep hoping that I'm that "one-in-a-million." He [the neurosurgeon] said it's very few that do get their feeling back and I'm hoping ... I'm lucky. I'm very lucky 'cause my arms and hands were never injured. His [a roommate who was quadraplegic] spine was severed, but I don't believe my spine was severed at all. I think my spine just got pinched.

I commented that he appeared to be thinking about the possibility that his spine was severed, a very real possibility. Nick continued,

I think probably if it's just pinched, my chances are a lot better of getting my legs back, than if it was severed. I know for a fact that if it was severed, I'll probably never get my legs back ... But then, the main thing is—if my spine was severed chances are very slim of my getting my legs back.

Nick explained how he planned to concentrate his "energy and will power" on his back every night before going to sleep in order to promote healing after surgery. I did not offer support for his plan, nor did I criticize it since he so obviously was using it as a means of coping.

During the fifth week Nick's anxiety had decreased in sharp contrast to its level on the previous Friday. He attempted to grasp the scope and objectives of later rehabilitation. His reference to another patient with a broken back seemed to reveal that he was still struggling to comprehend the "surprises" he encountered from his own injury. In addition to the young woman with the broken back, he was able to identify with a young roommate whose cervical spinal cord was severed. Nick even considered the possibility that his own spinal cord might be severed. He was able intermittently to analyze his fears of surgery, and absorbed preoperative and postoperative instructions.

At one time or another, Nick had at last confronted most of the threatening aspects in his situation. The combination of his realizations must have been so overwhelming that denial gradually ensued to help him cope. He could even become preoccupied with playing the guitar. Eventually, the impending surgery hardly bothered him and he could joke about it. He even concluded that he would only require two or three weeks of rehabilitation after getting off the Stryker frame. When Nick was again confronted with the fact that rehabilitation involved more than learning to use the wheelchair, his denial became almost defiant and adamant. He had already determined how he would continue to swim, fish, and enjoy nature whether "crippled or not." He was unwilling to believe that his injury could really change his life, except for hitchhiking. His boasting about his strength indicated an attempt to reestablish his previous self-identity. He appeared to inflate the possibility that he would not be permanently paralyzed; that he would be that "one in a million" who would walk again. He was very hopeful. If all else failed, he felt almost certain that concentrating his "energy and will power" on his back would enable him to walk again. This appeared to be an example of magical thinking or fantasy.

## WEEK 6

I arrived early Monday morning to provide Nick's nursing care before surgery. The night before, Nick had been transferred from the neurosurgical to the orthopedic patient care unit. Unfortunately neither I nor the nursing staff had anticipated the transfer and so Nick was not prepared for it. He reported that it made him angry and that he missed his previous roommate. Nick had been placed in a semiprivate room and he again had a young adult roommate. His parents had arrived on Sunday and were planning to stay until Tuesday. Nick revealed that he had not been hungry and had not eaten well on Sunday because he was "nervous." Several times he stated that he wished it were Tuesday so that his surgery would already be finished. Just before being transported to the operating room, Nick told his father, "I just keep thinking that I wouldn't be here today if I had listened to you and not gone hitchhiking."

During the surgical procedure Nick's spinal column was fused from the third through the seventh thoracic vertebrae. Nick tolerated the procedure quite well and was returned to his room in the afternoon. By the next morning he was taking oral fluids, but was still somewhat drowsy. After being medicated for pain in his back, he slept during most of the morning. His parents departed for home Tuesday evening after talking with a hospital social worker and Nick's surgeon. I had arranged the meeting with the social worker for Nick's parents to discuss the services available from Crippled Children's Services and how to apply.

By Friday Nick was comfortable, animated, and talkative. He stated that his surgery experience was not as bad as he thought it would be and he joked about having a sore throat since the operation. Nick appeared to be almost in an elated, euphoric state. He related the story of his accident and voiced his resentment of Bill, the driver of the car. "I probably never will hear from him and he better hope I don't see him again." Nick told how, since Thursday, he had again started to play his records and the guitar, and how he had "joked around and gave the nurses a bad time." He explained "I felt good yesterday, man, just like you doped me up again [referring to his preoperative medication]." He had also begun to identify as his new girlfriend a young hospital volunteer, Sandy, who was a college freshman. Sandy worked on her homework while visiting Nick in the evening and Nick described how he helped her. Although I doubted that Nick was that helpful to Sandy, I commented that he appeared to enjoy being with her.

Nick indicated that he had calculated how long he would have to remain in the hospital and that he hoped he would be able to go home for Christmas for a few days before entering a physical rehabilitation facility, probably Dodd Hall. He revealed that he had discussed with his father the problem of trying to keep his upstairs bedroom. Nick also displayed in his hospital room several photographs taken of himself playing the guitar while at home.

Nick avoided discussion of paralysis or changes in his future life. Also he did not ask questions about the outcome of his surgery. His ego-supportive boasting and the display of his photos seemed to indicate an attempt to reestablish his previous identity and console his damaged self-image.

## WEEK 7

During this second week after surgery Nick was very loquacious. He talked at length about his family, his hitchhiking trips and past girlfriends, and his attempts to start a rock music group. He stated he did not have the patience to start a new project in occupational therapy and instead just played his guitar and talked with the therapist.

His aunt had sent him a portable television and Nick and his roommate watched it nightly until after midnight. He again expressed his confidence that he could learn all he would need to know in two or three weeks at a rehabilitation facility. When informed that most paraplegic patients required several months of training, he replied, "Oh, I didn't think it would be *that* long." After learning that he could be fitted with a leg bag for urinary drainage, Nick said he liked to wear tight fitting "Levi's" and did not think the leg bag was a good idea. He had again discussed with his father the problem of his upstairs bedroom and the location for his rehabilitation and reported that he had manipulated the situation "so it seemed as if it was Dad's idea for me to stay at Dodd Hall." No definite decisions were made. Nick expressed some concern for his family's financial situation. I reminded him that some assistance for his rehabilitation might be obtained from his state's Crippled Childrens Service and Vocational Bureau of Rehabilitation.

Later Nick nonchalantly revealed that his roommate had told him two or three days after his surgery that Nick's spinal cord was severed. Nick explained that his roommate had overheard Nick's surgeons discussing this information. He then quickly changed the subject. He boasted about how he had "put the make on some student nurse" and joked about the nurses "just being real cool."

It was notable that since his surgery Nick no longer used the phrase "if I get my feeling back." He had been told by his roommate a few days after surgery that his spinal cord was severed, and the time of that incident corresponds to the euphoria which Nick experienced toward the end of the first week after surgery. Nick was aware that severing of the cord meant permanent disability. He seemed to negate what his roommate told him and did not even want to think about it. He was able to appear indifferent about his severed cord and his hunched back. His conversation focused on his past and the nonthreatening aspects of his life. He tended to avoid discussing his disability or the changes imposed by the disability. He appeared to reject the necessity for rehabilitation and the length of time it would require. Nick was unwilling to consider switching from his upstairs bedroom or abandoning his wish to wear tight-fitting trousers. His boasting and his denial of imposed changes appeared to be an attempt to rebuild his previous identity.

## WEEK 8

The stitches had been removed from Nick's back during the weekend. He had told his family about the possibility of being in Dodd Hall for two months. Nick commented, "I've already figured out a lot of ways to do a lot of things." He explained how he planned to get into the bathroom and bathtub using the wheelchair at home. He hoped to go home for a few days around Christmas. "I wanna go uptown. Like, a lot of my friends hang around town. Wheelchair or no wheelchair, ice or no ice [referring to the possibility of bad weather], I'm gonna get myself around town and see a lot of my friends." Nick's desire to see his peers is typical adolescent behavior as the peer group is very important in this stage of development.

Nick discussed how he perceived his physical condition. He said,

It's not actually . . . that I'm paralyzed . . but my spinal cord isn't hooked up right. I'm not actually paralyzed, I mean, paralyzed is when your spinal cord is not working. And my spinal cord is working. It's just not hooked up right . . . So, I'm not paralyzed actually . . . The nerves to my feet aren't connected to the nerves to my feet. Ya know, like my spinal cord was severed. And when they put them back together, they didn't make sure that the nerves to my feet were hooked up to the nerves to my feet, and that the nerves to my shins were hooked up to the nerves to my shins . . . and all that. They didn't put them back in place. It's like you take a telephone wire. It's got like, about close to 300 little wires in it—running through it. And if you cut one of those in half and then put it back together, not all those little wires are

going to go back together, and that's the same thing that
happened to me. My spinal cord is the telephone wire. Like if you
cut a telephone wire in half, you could take both ends and put
them back together again . . . But then if you twisted your hands
a little bit while you had it taken off and turned the wire slightly,
then you'd put it back together crooked . . . And if there was
anybody on the lines, they might get the wrong number. They
might be dialing one number and get another number . . . That's
about what happened to my spine. It got put back together
crooked.

When I asked from whom he had learned this information, Nick replied, "Nobody. It's just what I know about the
spinal cord. I mean I've studied human anatomy." I
explained that the spinal cord did not regenerate and
therefore no effort was made to rejoin the severed ends of his
spinal cord in surgery. He listened intently, then replied,

Now you've got me slightly confused. Do you remember when I
asked him [the neurosurgeon] about getting my legs back? He
said sometimes it does happen, but it's just a by-product of
surgery. So if it's a by-product of surgery, wouldn't those nerves
have to grow back together?

I explained that some return of function might occur,
but only in those instances where the spinal cord was not
severed. After a long pause, Nick asked, "Well, I don't think
mine was completely cut, was it?" I referred to the
information Nick had learned from an ex-roommate. Nick
replied,

Well, that's what Mike told me—that he heard a doctor say that
my spinal cord was severed. But like, I haven't asked any doctors
or anything. I don't know for a fact that it was severed. All I
know is that my back is broken—and out of wack . . . I'll ask my
doctor.

Nick then abruptly changed the subject.

During his morning care on Tuesday, Nick announced,
"I can feel the sun on my legs. It feels warm." I responded
that the sun was warm shining through the window into his

room. Later he revealed that he felt he was not really paralyzed because his internal organs were not affected—he still produced urine and feces. I explained that paralysis in this case referred to the loss of voluntary muscle control which he was experiencing. On Friday Nick learned that he would get off of the Stryker frame in about three weeks. He had received assurance from his orthopedic surgeon that he would be able to travel lying down on the back seat of the family car and could spend a few days at home around Christmas. He talked about the possibility of building wheel tracks on the stairs to his bedroom so that he could be pulled up to the room in a wheelchair.

Nick told about an ex-roommate who had visited him.

> He's confined to a wheelchair for a couple months, I guess. But that's not actually too long, ya know. He said he really hates the wheelchair, but I said, "Don't worry about it. I got one for life." . . . Well, a wheelchair will get me around and get me where I'm going and that's all that gonna count.

Nick again indicated his belief that he would not have to remain at Dodd Hall for very long. He had "figured out" how to dress himself. "But the main thing I'm gonna have to learn is how to work my bowels . . . Everything else I've already got figured out—at least to a certain extent." He said he now understood the reason for his transfer from the neurosurgical service to the orthopedic service because "evidently the ends of my spinal cord had died off and they figured they wouldn't be able to do anything with it." However, just a little later, he repudiated that statement.

> If my lungs hadn't been messed up the way they were . . . possibly I could've got my legs back. I just had to mess my lungs up when I hit that ground. It ruined everything . . . They could have fixed me up at least partially . . . because I don't actually believe my spinal cord was actually chopped right in two. I find that very hard to believe. Because the lump in my back went off to the right, but not that much to the right . . . 'Cause I saw the lump at night, ya know. When I had my light on, I could see my reflection

in the window. And I looked like a camel, ya know, and I could see the hump. And it didn't go that far to the right. So I find it hard to believe that my spinal cord was completely severed . . . Yet, that's what Mike [ex-roommate] said.

After a long pause he changed the subject. He had established the routine of calling home every Wednesday night because "it makes the week seems shorter." Nick thought he was keeping busy by reading, watching television, playing his guitar, and "spinning records." He explained that he had lost interest in occupational therapy and sometimes declined to go there. "It doesn't seem to take my mind off anything. It's like regular hospital routine and stuff."

During this eighth week of hospitalization Nick appeared to be struggling with the reality of his disability and at the same time denying the reality of his situation. His rather rigid denial during the previous week now appeared shaken. He was sporadically willing to reconsider and discuss some aspects of his situation. He began to think and plan on how to manage the activities of daily living as a paraplegic. Although his plans were not always reasonable, he began to make some short-term plans for his visit home at Christmas and also made reference to spending the rest of his life in a wheelchair. Some aspects of the reality of his situation were apparently unavoidable. At this time Nick began to use a future orientation in dealing with reality. This was interpreted as a superficial, but perhaps gradual, acknowledgment of his disability.

## WEEK 9

During this ninth week of his hospitalization Nick appeared to be peaceful and relaxed. He again stated that he did not think he would need to stay at Dodd Hall for two months because he already knew much about how to care for himself. His father had flu and was unable to visit over the weekend. Nick commented,

> He'd give his right arm to get up here to see me, but he was just too sick to come . . . I was his favorite son. I helped him with all the work he had to do, or most of it anyway—'cause I had all the muscles in the family—between me and Dad . . . I never bitched about any work that I had to do. Sometimes I'd forget to do it and I'd get in trouble for it, but I never bitched about it.

Nick's denial of past problems in his relationship with his parents appeared to be a coping mechanism. He boasted about how he had "cut" school and had written his own excuses for his absences. At times Nick's boasting was difficult to tolerate and I had to keep reminding myself that it was one of his means of coping. He discussed the part-time jobs he had held before his accident and remarked that he would not have any of them when he was discharged from the hospital. Nick hoped again to attempt to organize a rock music group when he returned home. To do this, he estimated that about one thousand dollars would be needed to buy new and additional equipment and he added, "but it really isn't that much." He thought that some day he might go to night school, but not day school because "the halls would be too crowded for a wheelchair to squeeze through." Nick stated that he wished he were thirty years old so that he would have had more years of "walking life" before he was paralyzed. He also said that he would not be in this position now if it were not for Bill, the driver of the car at the time of the accident. Nick expressed a desire to take vocational interest tests which were available at Dodd Hall and indicated he might be interested in a career in electronics. He also stated his hope that he could learn how to control his bowel movements if he could be at Dodd Hall a few days before going home for Christmas.

The data from this week seemed remarkable only when Nick's current tranquility was compared to his apparent anguish of the week before. His denial was apparently adequate to maintain comfort. He remained unwilling to accept the length of time necessary for rehabilitation.

**WEEK 10**

Nick was eager to progress with the preparations for using the wheelchair, such as being measured for a back brace and adjusting to an upright position. He was determined to tolerate being completely upright on his first day of using the tilt table. "I'm gonna stand straight. I'm gonna get up if it kills me." Nick related that he had felt pain traveling down his spine and that he had felt "a large piece of mucus" pass through his Foley catheter. During a Foley catheter change he reported that removal of the catheter felt as if his "intestines were being pulled out," though not actually *painful.*

In discussing his choice of a future vocation, Nick explained, "I think the main thing I like as a profession is my guitar. I mean, if it wasn't for my guitar I wouldn't have a thing to live for—except my family. And my guitar means so much to me—well, there was only one time that I offered to get rid of it." He had once offered to sell his guitar to help pay hospital expenses for his stepmother. He said, "Our family was never too cool on getting money. I'm 'Mister Rich' as far as our family goes. I'm the only one who can get money in our family." He again mentioned his interest in electronics and reported that two of his friends had taken apart a record player and could not put it back together again, but that he had assembled it in only two hours.

Some of this week's data appeared to be characteristic of the acknowledgment phase although the bulk of the data continued to be representative of defensive retreat. In referring to himself as a paraplegic, Nick appeared to have a shallow understanding of his situation. His disclosure that he had nothing to live for except his family and guitar seemed to reveal that self-depreciation had occurred. The reality of his disability had forced itself upon him at least to some extent as he became concerned for some of the aspects of his rehabilitation. He appeared to begin to deal with the reality of his situation in small fragments.

But denial still persisted to a great extent. Nick eagerly grasped and accepted the possibility that he could walk "with crutches." He continued to repudiate the duration and involvement of his rehabilitation. He even attempted to deny that his separation from family and friends involved an emotional expenditure. Nick maintained unrealistic vocational goals and appeared unwilling to plan logically for the future. He continued to experience vague periodic sensations below the level of his injury which implied rather obvious denial of his paralysis. He readily expressed his hostility toward the driver of the car at the time of the accident, perhaps in place of the hostility he could not express about his actual disability. His boasting persisted as an indication of his attempt to reestablish a previous identity.

## WEEK 11

Early in this week Nick explained that for a long time he had wanted a stereo tape recorder. He had not asked his parents to buy him the recorder because he knew that "they would have done anything to get it for me." But now his parents had bought him the recorder he wanted for Christmas. He analyzed their action in terms of his relationship with his parents.

> In our family, my dad likes me best of all the kids. It's not just like all the other kids are rats—but I can help him when he has to have work done . . . I was the guy who would always go with him 'cause I was the one with the muscles. And, like, most of the time, I could outwork Dad in anything I knew how to do, ya know . . . So, I was more or less the favorite son and a lot of times him and Ma both told me so.

Nick had received a letter from a school friend in response to a letter he had written earlier. "I told her, 'Next time you see me, I'll be in a real live genuine wheelchair.' She wrote that whether I'm in a wheelchair or not, I'd still be the same old Nick. She remembered me as I used to be and not as I am. That was real encouraging 'cause we've been friends for so long." Nick explained that he had gone to school with this girl for eight years and that he had used her hair pins to shoot from a rubber band. He said he was an expert shot and had taught this "skill" to some of his friends. When a roommate's visitor asked what had happened to him, Nick readily replied, "I broke my back in an auto accident . . . I'm paralyzed from here on down (pointing to mid-chest) and I can't feel anything."

Again Nick voiced his intention to attain a vertical position on his first day of using the tilt table. He even thought he would be able to walk upstairs using braces. "I don't think I'll have any problem walking upstairs. I'll admit I'm paralyzed way up to here (points to mid-chest) and my feeling stops—and I'm paralyzed from here down . . . But still I think I can make it up the stairs. I'll do it. I'm determined."

Later, on hearing a small child crying in the hall, Nick said, "I'd like to have kids some day, but I know I won't be able to now. Maybe by artificial insemination I could." He thought he would not be able to have intercourse, but thought intercourse might be possible for a paraplegic who did not need or could remove a catheter. Nursing personnel caring for Nick reported to me that recently Nick made frequent references to sexual functioning, to past sexual "conquests" and that he occasionally attempted to pat or rub the legs of young female personnel. I encouraged these personnel to be very direct in dealing with aspects of Nick's behavior to which they took offense. I cautioned them to direct their comments specifically to his behavior and not in a general way to Nick as a person. I also had noticed Nick's apparent increasing concern for his future sexual functioning.

Christopherson contends that the primary biologic sex role is a part of the integrated male ego. Sex problems arising with some frequency in disabled males are impotence, lack of sex partners, and physical or emotional barriers to sexual activity. The significance of sexual adequacy plays an important part in the total adjustment of disabled individuals.[5]    For the disabled male adolescent adjustment is extremely difficult because the period of adolescence is when the male libido is at its peak. Likewise, the individual's masculinity is measured often by his adolescent peer group according to the number of sexual conquests he has achieved. Sexual conformity is very important during the adolescent period. Rejection of the adolescent with a disability is most likely to occur in groups, because in them the myth of the ideal physique is most relevant. This is particularly true in the area of courtship and marriage where rigid conformity is demanded in sex appropriateness. The adolescent with a disability is convinced that his difficulties in heterosexual relationships would be obliterated were it not for his disability. It should be helpful for him to know that physical conformity will not always be so essential to sex appropriateness, and that for most persons with disabilities, courtship and marriage are not forever barred, though they are often delayed.[3]

Since Nick was able to have at least a reflex erection, I discussed with him the probability that he would be able to have intercourse but be unable to have children. Nick said he realized that he probably would not be able to experience orgasm but would find satisfaction in being able to have intercourse. According to Zeitlin, Cottrell, and Lloyd the higher the disabled male's spinal lesion, the more probable is the occurrence of a satisfactory erection, as reflection erections are mediated through the sacral portion of the spinal cord.[6] However, the male is often sterile after spinal cord injury due to failure of spermatogenesis, obstruction of genital passages as a result of frequent infection, or neuromuscular dysfunction, particularly failure to ejaculate.[7]

When I arrived Friday, Nick was lying on his back with
an arm thrown across his eyes and a pillow partially covering
his head. He said he was angry, very angry. He had been
fitted with a back brace on Wednesday. Since he now had the
brace, he wanted to begin using the tilt table today although
he was not scheduled to do so until the following Monday.
He wanted to be up in the wheelchair when his parents
arrived on Saturday. Nick said he felt that his physician had
avoided him today because "he knew what I wanted." He felt
the food and the "service" were poor and he was "tired of
the whole damn hospital." He stated that he already knew
how to get from his bed into a wheelchair and that he could
progress "a hell of a lot faster than what they're taking me."
Nick was sullen, his voice quivered, and he swore frequently.
I tried to be a nonjudgmental, nondefensive listener while
Nick ventilated his angry feelings related to his dependent
status.

The data from this week indicated that Nick continued
to vacillate between denial and acknowledgment of his
situation. He readily described himself as being paralyzed,
even to a complete stranger. In discussing his correspondence
from a school friend, Nick appeared to be concerned about
acceptance by his peers now that he was disabled. He was
beginning to think what his disability would mean for him in
the future. He had thought about his potential for sexual
activity and he appeared to be considering the effect that his
disability would have on his self-image and male role.

Nick's denial was predominant, although concomitant
with the acknowledgment of his circumstances. His boasting
and his description of his relationship with his parents
appeared again to be an attempt to reaffirm his previous
identity and status. His reference to being a strong and able
worker seemed to imply reluctance to change his image of
self and body. The data from Friday indicated that Nick was
angered at being unable to control the events of his life. He
freely expressed his hostility toward his physician and the
hospital. And he was defiant in his denial of his disability.

Although still confined to the Stryker frame, Nick felt certain that he would be able to use braces, that he could already transfer into a wheelchair by himself, and that he could progress much faster with physical activity if allowed to do so.

## WEEK 12

On Monday Nick was again calm and dispassionate. He had been transferred from the Stryker frame to a regular bed on Sunday. He had been placed on the tilt table several times on Monday and had been able to tolerate being elevated to 65 degrees for seven to eight minutes. He threatened to "beat up" Bill, the accident driver, and struck his fist on the overhead trapeze on his bed as he talked. With his transfer to a rehabilitation center perhaps only one week away, he was undecided about whether to go to Dodd Hall or to a location nearer his home. "There are two things I wanna do. I would like to stay here with my friends, but I also wanna help my parents. And I would rather help my parents than stay with my friends." His parents had told him that if he were nearer home, their visits would be more frequent and less expensive than if he were to stay in Columbus. He commented, "A seat belt is something I should have been wearing before the accident, then I wouldn't have had to spend twelve weeks in the hospital and two months in a rehabilitation center."

On Tuesday Nick was again placed on the tilt table in physical therapy and was able to tolerate a vertical position. He was then assisted into a wheelchair for the first time. He smiled proudly as he wheeled himself back to his room and stopped frequently to greet patients and personnel that he knew. His orthopedic surgeon told Nick that he could be discharged as soon as arrangements could be made for his rehabilitation. When Nick called his parents to discuss the arrangements, they decided that Nick would remain in the hospital until the day before Christmas, and then go to a rehabilitation center nearer his home.

But by Friday the plans were changed. Nick announced, "I get to go to Dodd Hall Monday or Tuesday [of the following week]. I get to go home Wednesday!" He and his parents decided that Nick would return to Dodd Hall after the Christmas weekend and that perhaps "later" he would be transferred to a rehabilitation facility nearer their home. Nick stated that he was sometimes embarrassed by his lack of bowel control and viewed this as a goal of his rehabilitation. Yet he continued to believe that his rehabilitation would not take long.

The data from this last week of the study indicated that Nick was still primarily experiencing denial of his situation. He continued to express his hostility toward Bill and threatened to beat him, a threat he obviously could not carry out. He boasted about how much he already would know when he arrived at a rehabilitation facility and was persistent in refusing to acknowledge the duration and involvement of his rehabilitation. He also had difficulty in making final plans for his rehabilitation, perhaps because he was unable to accept the need for them. This, however, is also characteristic of adolescents, as they typically have difficulty making decisions to which they can adhere. In addition, Nick appeared to be concentrating on his physical progress.

Nick's comment regarding his not wearing a seat belt at the time of the accident seemed to indicate more acknowledgment of his own responsibility in the accident. He continued to identify bowel training as a rehabilitation concern. He attempted to consider his parents, as well as his own desires, in selecting a rehabilitation facility, although the final choice appeared to be in compromise. In all, Nick appeared to be willing to consider only small fragments of the harsh reality of his situation at any one time.

## SUMMARY

I found the 12-week period of caring for Nick to be very rewarding and satisfying. Although at times the experience was emotionally draining for me, I was impressed with the tremendous amount of effort and strength Nick displayed as he attempted to deal with the impact of his disability. I felt I had shared a difficult experience with him to some extent and that our relationship hopefully made his situation easier for him.

Nick's life experiences prior to his injury greatly influenced his becoming a very unique and interesting adolescent. Though unique as an individual, Nick's psychosocial needs were very typical of a sixteen-year-old normal adolescent male, and he was struggling with the problems of personal identity, emotional independence, authority, and peer socialization. His struggle became much more difficult following his sudden physical disability and hospitalization. Nick's disability posed a great threat to his sex role and sexual adequacy; to his ability to meet the adolescent culture's demands for conformity in physique, dress, and behavior; and to his preparation for economic independence.

## EPILOGUE

Nick spent only 5 weeks at Dodd Hall before being transferred to a rehabilitation facility in his home state. Thereafter, I had only periodic communication from him by mail. Rehabilitation was a very difficult experience for Nick as the months passed. He apparently presented rehabilitation personnel with many challenges. Approximately a year and a half after his accident, Nick wrote from home that he was relatively independent with the aid of a wheelchair and that he was planning to enroll in an electronics training program sponsored by his state's Bureau of Vocational Rehabilitation.

## REFERENCES

1. Schonfeld WA: Body image in adolescents: a psychiatric concept for the pediatrician. Pediatrics, Vol 31, May 1963, pp 845–46, 851
2. Gunther MS: Emotional aspects. In Ruge D (ed): Spinal Cord Injuries. Springfield, Ill, Charles C Thomas, 1969, p 97
3. Wright BA: Physical Disability: A Psychological Approach. New York, Harper, 1960, pp 118, 179–81
4. Havighurst RJ: Developmental Tasks and Education, 2nd ed. New York, McKay, 1952, pp 2, 4, 33–71
5. Christopherson V: Role modification of the disabled male. Am J Nurs, Vol 68, Feb 1968, pp 290–93
6. Zeitlin AB, Cottrell T, Lloyd FA: Sexology of the paraplegic male. Fertil Steril, Vol 8, July–Aug 1957, pp 337–44
7. Talbot HS: The sexual function in paraplegia. J Urol, Vol 73, Jan 1955, pp 91–100

## BIBLIOGRAPHY

Aguilera DC, Messick JM, Farrell MS: Crisis Intervention: Theory and Methodology. St Louis, Mosby, 1970

Christopherson V: Role modification of the disabled male. Am J Nurs, Vol 68, Feb 1968

Gunther MS: Emotional aspects. In Ruge D (ed): Spinal Cord Injuries, Springfield, Ill, Charles C Thomas, 1969

Havighurst RJ: Developmental Tasks and Education, 2nd ed. New York, McKay, 1952

Morley WE, Messick JM, Aguilera DC: Crisis: paradigms of intervention. J Psychiatr Nurs, Vol 5, 1967

Ruge D (ed): Spinal Cord Injuries. Springfield. Ill, Charles C Thomas, 1969

Schonfeld WA: Body image in adolescents: a psychiatric concept for the pediatrician. Pediatrics, Vol 31, May 1963

Shontz FC: Reactions to crisis. Volta Review, Vol 67, 1965

———: Severe chronic illness. In Garrett JF, Levine ES (eds): Psychological Practice with the Physically Disabled. New York, Columbia U Press, 1962

Talbot HS: The sexual function in paraplegia. J Urol, Vol 73, Jan 1955

Wacks H, Zaks M: Studies of body image in men with spinal cord injuries. J Nerv Ment Dis, Vol 131, 1960

Wright BA: Physical Disability: A Psychological Approach. New York, Harper, 1960

Zeitlin AB, Cottrell T, Lloyd FA: Sexology of the paraplegic male. Fertil Steril, Vol 8, July–Aug 1957

# 9

# Adolescent Suicide and the Suicidal Adolescent

KAY FORSYTHE FENTON

In this chapter I will discuss what I consider to be two separate issues—adolescent suicide and the suicidal adolescent. A review of the literature shows that suicide and suicidal attempts are more common in children and adolescents than is generally realized. Many suicides and suicide attempts are not reported as such but are classified as accidents. Accidents lead all other causes of death in children and adolescents.

Adolescence is a turbulent and critical period of growth and development, and so physicians, teachers, parents, and others concerned with the welfare of adolescents must learn to recognize danger signals in youngsters who might later attempt suicide if help is not provided. Some danger signals are "sudden change in behavior and personality, irritability, depression, ready unprovoked agitation, anxiety, outbursts of temper, threat or mild attempt at suicide, insomnia, love fallouts, change in mood, anorexia, and poor parent-child relationships. Early detection of the potential suicide, the 'suicide prone,' and prompt referral for indicated care may avert many needless tragedies."[1]

## ADOLESCENT SUICIDE

At any age suicide is an act of desperation. Suicide is the eighteenth leading cause of death in the 10- to 14-year-old group and the fifth leading cause of death in persons age 15 to 19 in the United States. In suicide, "there is an element of conscious intention which is not present in the other 'accidents.' "[2]

In the 10- to 14-year-old group the suicide rate among boys is 6 times greater than for girls. Most articles indicated that suicides in this age range are impulsive and do not manifest the characteristics of suicidal attempts of later adolescents or adults. "They are immature, impulsive young-sters who react excessively to stress, often of a minor nature."[3] Precipitating factors could be an unhappy home, fear of punishment, difficulty in school, and/or injured pride. These adolescents usually come from homes broken by divorce, separation, abandonment, or death of a parent. Their motives are rebellion against the parents, lack of parental affection, protest against restriction of liberty, fear of imprisonment after antisocial acts, unhappiness in love, jealousy, wounded pride. The child's size and ego status are against his use of specific instruments of destruction. "Suicide in children has multiple motivations, but the primary dynamic reason is the real or threatened loss of a love object."[4] The child is dependent on the love object and the process of identification is not complete. The turning of hostility inward and destroying the introjects within themselves are painful and frightening. Their self-destructive feelings are expressed by accidental injuries which can result in the destruction of the individual. These accidents are "desperate attempts at regaining contact with the lost gratifying love object."[4](p 132)

There is a sharp increase in suicides in the 15- to 19-year-old range. The male-female ratio in this age range is 3 to 1. Firearms and explosives are the most common means used by adolescents in the United States to commit suicide. Hanging and strangulation in boys and poisoning in girls are the next most commonly utilized means. "Self-destruction is rare under 10 years and remains infrequent until 15 years of age, when a sharp rise in both boys and girls takes place. The rate continues to increase in boys throughout the 15- to 19-year age period; the rate for girls shows an upward trend during these years."[2](pp 752-53)

Multiple factors usually lead the adolescent to a point where he sees no other way to handle his problem except through suicide. "The outstanding element seems to be a vulnerable personality which is unable to meet everyday life experiences and everyday problems in an integrated, understanding, and effective manner."[2](p 766) These adolescents seem ill equipped to cope with problems owing to inadequate homes, parental indifference, or rejection, and lack of cooperation between school and home. Among the personal factors which predispose an adolescent to suicide are physical defects producing feelings of inferiority, hormonal change accompanying adolescence, anxiety associated with pubertal changes, realization of some sexual abnormality, sex contacts and experiences, difficulty in social adjustment, a hereditary or familial weakness, personality disorders, psychosis, and low intelligence. Predisposing features in the environment could be a home broken by divorce, separation, or death, unaffectionate parents, neglect, mental instability of members in the home, friction with siblings, feelings of exclusion, a feeling of being unwanted, school difficulty, or friction with teachers or schoolmates. The adolescent is more capable than the child of hurting himself because he is physically an adult and he is less dependent on the love object.

There are certain generalizations concerning suicide that hold throughout the life cycle. "Suicide is more common in males than in females and in whites than in nonwhites. Urban dwellers outnumber rural, and professional groups [and students] outnumber workers."[2(p 759)]The overall suicide rate fluctuates according to the season of the year, declining during summer and autumn and rising during winter, reaching its highest point around May. A strong influence on the incidence of suicide is exerted by religious affiliation. Personal problems are more fully resolved the firmer the church organization and the more devoted the members to their beliefs. There also are external causes for suicide which have to do with the social milieu. The suicide rate rises in times of social disturbances and economic crises. These external factors affect the incidence of suicides in children and adolescents more than in adults.

Parents of adolescent suicides need help in going through the grieving process and in completing the grieving process. "Death is always distressing to relatives and friends who remain behind, but it is especially so in the case of suicide, for here grief is accompanied by shame and by feelings of guilt and inadequacy. Most parents feel that they are in some way responsible for the unhappiness which expressed itself in this extreme fashion."[2(p767)]Most parents have difficulty understanding adolescent behaviors and dealing with them. Self-destruction is particularly hard to understand. "The voluntary act of taking one's own life represents a failure in communication between the individual and his meaningful object relationships, together with an inability to cope with the stresses of life."[5]

## THE SUICIDAL ADOLESCENT

Suicidal behavior, either threatened or attempted, should be taken very seriously. The suicidal adolescent communicates his self-destructive intent through sharing suicidal thoughts, threats, plans, gestures, and suicidal attempts. "The person considering suicide is always ambivalent—he wishes to live at the same time he wishes to die—and because suicide is a cry for help, the potential victim will almost always signal his intention."[6]

Attempted suicide in adolescents is common; the ratio of attempted suicides to actual suicides is in the magnitude of 100:1. Suicidal attempts of adolescents represent a large percentage of the total attempts by any age group, about 12 percent. There is a marked increase in attempts in the 15 to 19 age group over the 10 to 14 age group. All articles in the literature pointed to the large increase of females who attempt suicide in the 15 to 19 group. The female adolescent in the 15 to 19 age group represents over 90 percent of the total number of suicide attempts at this age. A reason for the high incidence of suicidal attempts in the adolescent, particularly the female, is probably due to impulsiveness. The attempt is not truly a premeditated act, nor does the individual actually desire or intend to die.

"One of the reasons that suicidal attempts have been overlooked in children and adolescents is the erroneous concept that youngsters do not experience depression."[3 (p 721)]They do not exhibit the signs and symptoms of adult depression reactions but other symptoms instead. "In latency the child exhibits behavioral problems [temper tantrums, disobedience, truancy, feelings that no one cares for him, running away from home, accident proneness, masochistic actions, self-destructive behavior] which often indicate depressive feelings."[3 (p 722)] The child is convinced that he is bad, evil, unacceptable and these feelings lead him into antisocial behavior which further reinforces his belief that he is no good. He feels inferior to other children, often that he is ugly and stupid. In addition, boys have a need to hide soft, tender, weak sentiments. The child often uses denial to ward off depressive feelings.

The adolescent can exhibit his depression by boredom, restlessness, and/or a preoccupation with trivia. He loses interest in things, constantly seeks new ways to entertain himself, cannot stand to be alone, must be constantly busy, and needs continual stimulation to escape boredom. The adolescent may use acting out by means of delinquency, sexual promiscuity, use of alcohol and drugs to escape his depressive feelings. Other signs of depression in adolescents are excessive fatigue, hypochondriacal preoccupation, difficulty in concentration, insomnia, instability, and violent temper outbursts.

The suicidal attempt in most cases is a "sudden precipitous reaction to a stressful situation resulting from frustration, depression, overt or masked anger, or as a rebellious act against a restraining figure, a loved one."[1](p 103) The adolescent uses the suicidal attempt to frighten, to cause restraining persons to have a change of attitude or behavior toward him, to warn parents, to express dissatisfaction or displeasure with existing unpleasant situations, and as a plea to improve relationships.

Toolan uses five categories to classify the causes of suicidal attempts.

1. Anger at another which is internalized in the form of guilt and depression. Usually this anger is at the parents.
2. Attempts to manipulate another, to gain love and affection, to punish another. These are often directed at the parents with the fantasy that the parents will feel bad when the adolescent is dead. Adolescent girls use this when rejected by their boyfriends.
3. A signal of distress. The attempt is a dramatic and last ditch effort to call attention to one's problems hoping that help will come.

4. Reactions to feelings of inner disintegration, as a response to hallucinatory commands, as a desire for peace and a nirvana-like existence.
5. A desire to join a dead relative may appear of importance.[3]

Attempted suicides are of universal occurrence and are not limited to any social, economic, or racial group. The family of the suicidal adolescent frequently shows a high incidence of family disorganization. "There is evidence that the breaking up of a home creates for the child emotional traumata and unresolved conflicts that may lead to an inability to cope with loss in later life and predispose to the development of depressive reactions culminating in suicidal behavior."[7] The parents of suicidal youngsters tend to demonstrate an intense degree of ambivalence toward them, often weighted heavily in the direction of unconscious resentment, hostility, and rejection.

Sabbath talks about the concept of the expendable child to account for one of the multiple factors contributing to adolescent suicidal behavior. The onset of adolescence is called the "escalation stage" where an intensification of past behavioral problems between child and parent takes place. Past efforts of the parents to control their child's behavior and contain their own ambivalent feelings toward him begin to fail. The adolescent's continuing provocative behavior, changeable moods, periods of withdrawal, and secretiveness add to the parent's feeling of helplessness, frustration, and of being shut out. "Now another form of communication, of a different order, comes through: the nonverbal and unconscious kind that gives a message to the adolescent of his being no longer wanted: of his parent's [or parents'] wish to be rid of him and for him to die."[5 (p 282)] The child picks up the clues from his parents which can be communicated nonverbally as well as verbally, unconsciously as well as consciously, and may try to follow his parents' unconscious (or conscious) wishes and attempt suicide to gain their approval and love. The expendable child is the one who is no longer tolerated or needed by his family. He is no longer useful either as an object of affection or as the vicarious source of fulfilling the needs of his parents. He becomes the scapegoat, that is, the object through whom the parents deal with family and personal tensions. The adolescent feels that he should be dispensed with for the sake of everyone's welfare and reacts by attempting suicide. "There is much evidence from research that has been done that there is severe disturbance in the early childhood of suicidal adolescents in terms of parent-child relations and that this tends to become more pronounced in the adolescent period in terms of severe communication gaps within the family of suicidal adolescents."[8]

Suicidal attempts in adolescents are influenced by the season of the year. An increased incidence occurs during the spring (April–June); the next highest incidence during January–March; the highest incidence occurs in the month of May, and the lowest in September.

"Though most of the attempts at suicide are of an impulsive nature and resulting from a temporary emotional upset and not a desire to die, they may end fatally due to a miscalculation and from delay in obtaining prompt and appropriate treatment. Every attempt must be taken seriously and every individual who has made an attempt at suicide or who has threatened it should be referred for indicated psychiatric and medical help with a view towards determining the underlying influencing factors responsible for the act."[1 (p 104)]

## THE HOSPITALIZED SUICIDAL ADOLESCENT

"Treatment of any kind of suicidal behavior must begin with an evaluation of the seriousness of a child's suicidal desires. Observing the child, interviewing his parents, and examining the environment, should enable an investigator to determine whether a child presents a significantly dangerous risk. Glaser (1965) offers some criteria to be appraised: depth of the conflict, inner resources for coping with the situation, outer resources available, and severity of the stressful situation."[9] "Many therapists feel that unless the diagnostic picture suggests an overwhelming likelihood of imminent suicide, most cases of attempted suicide should be managed within the family."[10] Home management includes three areas which require attention.

1. sterilization of the physical home environment, and clearing the home of all easily available lethal materials.
2. parental therapy, which is basically supportive
3. direct therapy with the adolescent

In direct therapy, not only is there a need to make a quick and firm relationship with the therapist, who must be giving, but also, as soon as possible, the therapist must give interpretations so that the child can understand his own behavioral motivations.

Shochet talks about the administration of first aid by a physician to the potential suicide. He suggests the following: (1) Form a relationship with the patient to try to give the patient hope. This is done by trying to clarify, not to kindly reassure or to criticize; (2) be able to accept what is revealed—make the patient feel understood by discussing what matters; (3) attack the isolation of the patient; enlist the cooperation of family and friends; (4) involve the family as soon as possible in planning for the patient, just as would be the case in any medical emergency; (5) make a definite return appointment; (6) insist on psychiatric hospitalization if safety is in doubt; (7) give only small doses of medication especially if suicide is a definite possibility.[9(p 41)]

Immediate precautions must be taken for children who are identified as high risk. High risk suicide groups are defined as depressed patients, the chronically ill and isolated, bereaved patients, the disoriented or delirious, patients with a history of previous suicide attempts or previous suicide threats, those with current verbal or behavioral declarations of suicidal intent, patients displaying situations or syndromes conducive to suicidal response, and those with a family history of suicide. Hospitalization is the most effective precautionary measure. Shaw and Schelkun (1965) set forth some of the advantages of temporarily hospitalizing the child: (1) it provides a "breathing" spell for both child and family; (2) it removes the child from all stressful or anxiety-producing situations; (3) it allows the child to be observed and evaluated; (4) it indicates to the child that he is being helped, and that his problems are being taken seriously; and (5) it enables the child to accept a therapeutic relationship more easily.[11]

When the patient is admitted to the hospital the nurse who admits the patient to the unit should, if possible, be the nurse who will follow the patient throughout his hospitalization. She should let him know that she will be spending time with him daily and that she is concerned about him. The admitting nurse should give her patient a good deal of personal attention to help combat his feelings of hopelessness and isolation. She should make an assessment of the patient's condition, physical as well as mental, to obtain and record baseline data. This assessment should include identifying information such as: name, sex, age, who the patient lives with; the patient's mental status, including his state of consciousness, his orientation, attention span, intellectual capacity, and his suicidal ideation; the patient's physical status including his eyes, buccal cavity, state of skin and appendages, his sensory perception, nutritional state, elimination, state of physical rest and comfort, motor ability, and dress; the patient's emotional/behavior status including mood, presence or absence of anxiety, self-image, ability to relate to others, and so forth, his response to hospitalization, and the nurse's impressions of him. "He should be asked directly whether he has any suicidal means secreted about his person, and his possessions should be carefully searched but always with an attempt to keep this from being a degrading experience."[11](p 300)

It is important that the nurse help the patient feel comfortable on the unit. The unit routine should be explained carefully and time should be allowed for the patient to ask questions. The patient should be introduced to the other nurses and attendants. He should also be introduced to other patients as well. "The newly admitted patient must not be allowed to drift off alone or sit in his room unattended. A private room is to be avoided. When possible, a special nurse can be extremely supportive and protective for the first few days; for the highest-risk patients, continuous observation is imperative. Above all, the new patient must know exactly to whom to go if he feels in need, and he must not be given the notion that he is bothering the nurses and doctors with the demands."[11](p 300)

The presence or absence of strict suicidal precautions in hospitals varies widely from entirely open hospital settings where few precautions are possible to tight security cells. "Neither of these extremes is suitable. The best precaution against suicide in a hospital is the combination of an alert, well-trained staff, and the removal of easy temptations from those patients who are the most likely to commit suicide."[12] Razors, scissors, lighters, and plastic bags should not be readily available on a unit. If a patient is extremely suicidal, intent on harming himself with anything possible, the staff may have to remove glass containers, belts, and the like from his environment. With more staff contact and observation, the freedom of choice of a suicide method is greatly reduced and there is a need for greater ingenuity on the part of the patient to devise methods by which he can make a suicide attempt. This involves either the utilization of supposedly innocuous objects or methods to evade the control of staff.

For the patient determined to take his life, the environment is obviously filled with potential tools that cannot be removed from his reach. For example, head ramming, asphyxia by aspiration of paper, asphyxia by food, and exsanguination by tearing blood vessels with fingers, "these all are constantly available to the patient and only careful attention can prevent their use."[11](p 299)

Each hospital should have an area where withdrawn, psychotic, or deeply depressed and agitated patients can be confined and closely observed. This area in the hospital in which I work is called the "special care" unit. The patient is observed and the observations are recorded every 15 minutes or sooner if the staff feels closer observation is necessary. Sometimes we stay in the special care unit with the patient until he is calmer. He may be given medication to help him calm down. It is important that the patient not be confined to this area any longer than is absolutely necessary. Physical limits placed on the patient are merely substitutes for close staff supervision of the patient. Usually the better the training of the nursing staff, the less the patient will need to be confined.

The inpatient treatment should be conducted by a trained and coordinated clinical staff. "It is essential that the suicidal patient have a therapist in attendance who is managing the treatment, who is available to the patient within a reasonably short time, and who is not in conflict with the rest of the clinical staff. Fear, hesitation, confusion, or disagreement among the members of the staff is distinctly harmful to the suicidal patient. [The patient can see the staff's division and therefore feels less secure and more hopeless and may become more suicidal.] The therapist must also develop a relationship with the significant members of the patient's family at an early stage in the therapy, to bring to the family an awareness of the patient's distress and to facilitate resumption of open communication within the family unit."[11](p 301)

Early in treatment the therapist must help the youngster to realize the seriousness of his situation, but he must be careful to avoid premature interpretations that may only frighten the youngster away from therapy. The child must feel that he can trust the therapist in order to face his depressive problems. If he can not, he may avoid therapy and use avoidance, denial, and acting out to escape from his painful feelings. He may test the therapist to see if he cares for him and loves him. "Psychotherapy in the hospital should be viewed as the initial phase of a longer process that will lead the patient to an understanding of his problems, a constructive reordering of his life, and a strengthening of his identity."[9](p 42)

Group therapy can be of value to some patients. It should, however, supplement but not replace individual therapy.

Depressed children and adolescents usually do not benefit to the same degree from electro-convulsive therapy as do depressed adults. However, several authors reported the successful use of antidepressive drugs in treating young people. "Even the best psychopharmalogical agents are not considered to be the final answer, since the general belief is that medication is not as effective in children as in adults, and that medication alone is not effective treatment—only psychotherapy for both the child and his family, can lead to a permanent cure."[11](p 303)

It is important that all personnel in contact with the patient work together as a team. The patient will come in contact with many different staff members while in the hospital. The physician is usually responsible for all therapeutic decisions and usually correlates the functioning of the staff. All staff members coming in contact with the patient need to be kept informed on details and any changes in therapy. Occupational therapy, recreational therapy, and educational therapy (school programs) are also vital to a rich hospital program. "The staff should in general strive to develop a program which will prevent the suicidal patient from becoming fixed in his masochistic, self-pitying, resentful, isolated state."[13]

The nurse should have authority to make decisions

concerning the patient's daily management. The nursing staff will have the most contact with the patient while he is in the hospital. They will have to evaluate the patient daily or even hourly to determine his mood, what type of activities are appropriate, and what precautions if any are necessary. The nurse must know where the suicidal patient is, what he is doing, and observe him closely; he may try to leave the unit to carry out his intentions so he must be watched closely for this. The nurse might have to restrain the patient physically so he cannot carry out his destructive impulses. She can often anticipate this behavior by observing the patient for increased tension, anxiety, rapid mood swings, withdrawing from others, and being secretive. "Vigilance should not be relaxed as the patient seemingly improves. This period is one in which suicide is more apt to occur. As the patient's depression lifts and he begins to gain more insight, his anxiety may increase temporarily. Then, too, he may be only masking his true feelings so that he will be given more leeway to carry out his former threats."[13(p 201)] The nurse must evaluate the individual patient daily, using the information she gains from her observations and interactions with him to make decisions as to the plan of care for that day.

The nurse-patient relationship with the suicidal youngster is not easily established. "The nurse must have a genuine interest in the patient and must really want to help him. As the nurse empathizes with the patient, she will reflect a mood and attitude which is in harmony with his in that it will not be overly cheerful, but she will be warm, calm, serious, kind, and understanding."[14] The nurse should speak to the patient and spend time with him even though he may not respond. She should increase gradully the time she spends with the patient. One element in establishing a relationship with the patient is increasing his opportunities for communication with the nurse. Communication is verbal (talking, corresponding) and nonverbal (gesturing, physical contact). The nurse *must* establish and maintain communication with the patient. "Since communication is a two-way arrangement, we must be concerned with the content of two sets of messages—those we receive from the child and those we communicate to the child."[14(p 66)]

One way a youngster communicates is through his behavior. The nurse must be sensitive to what this behavior can tell of the child's hidden feelings. She must develop an awareness of the sometimes subtle and partially hidden messages that are contained in the youngster's behavior. For example, the youngster may be very secretive with the other patients and the nurse may feel that he may be going to try to hurt himself. She should talk with him about her feelings and try to find out what his mood is. She should observe him very closely until she again feels comfortable with him.

The youngster's behavior when he first comes into the hospital will be restrained. Not being sure what will happen to him, he manages temporarily to hold in check many of those behaviors that caused him to be admitted to the hospital. After he has oriented himself, he will begin to test his limits; the suicidal patient may try to hurt himself. The way the nurse handles this situation may encourage further interaction with the patient or alienate him. The nurse should look upon any confrontations as an important opportunity to communicate to the patient that she is somehow different from many adults with whom the patient has previously had encounters. She must deal with limit-testing behavior in a straightforward, firm, but unexcited manner.

The adolescent usually experiences what Erikson calls "basic mistrust." "Unlike normal children, these children have not learned to associate adults with pleasant experiences; they have not found that adults meet their needs in predictable ways, nor can adults be counted on in time of trouble."[14(p 71)] Youngsters may react to those feelings of mistrust in several different ways. First, they may withdraw, avoiding interaction with the nurse. The youngster should not be pursued too closely, but gradually should get to know the nurse. Second, the adolescent may try to disarm the nurse for, if he gets the upper hand, he need not fear the adult as strongly. For example, the youngster may claim he knows something about the nurse and is going to tell her boss. Or, he may attack the nurse. If the youth's experiences have taught him that adults are dangerous and should not be trusted, then he is apt to be somewhat confused when his experience with the nursing staff member does not bear this out. He may try to prove that the adult is untrustworthy. For example, he will try to catch the nurse in a lie or provoke a fight with her. A third stratagem the adolescent may try is camouflage. "By camouflaging his interest in the adult under seemingly hostile or frivolous behavior he can both maintain some communication and further test out the safety of the adult. If the adult misinterprets the child's behavior he may cause the child to abandon further communication."[14 (p 71)]

In addition, the teenager may have trouble trusting the nurse simply because some youngsters feel adults cannot be trusted. "If the trust barrier is to be removed, the child must learn that the adults are concerned with his welfare rather than with deceiving or exploiting him. This distrust is why it is so important that the adult always be honest in his dealings with children."[14 (p 94)]

In communicating verbally with the patient the nurse may encourage and reassure him by talking with him on neutral topics or simply by making small talk. Gradually the youth will begin to talk, and the nurse can then become an attentive listener. She will let him know that she is interested in what he says by occasional comments. By no means should the nurse ever cut off the patient's communication with her about his suicidal ideas because of her own feelings. As he gains insight into his problems through psychotherapy, the youth will gradually take more interest in himself and in those about him. The nurse can then gradually withdraw some of her attention from him and act as a catalyst in enhancing his relationships with others.

The nurse must communicate her observations and interactions with the patient to all those concerned with his care. It is important that the nurse's notes be written clearly so that the therapist can follow what is happening with the patient on the unit. In addition, she must communicate verbally with the therapist to express her concerns, ask questions, and develop a plan of care for the patient.

Together the staff must decide when the patient is ready for discharge. All staff members should be able to express their opinion and a decision should be reached. It is important that follow-up care be provided after discharge. "Perhaps more common than in hospital suicide is suicide immediately or shortly after discharge."[15] The therapist should inform the patient about the resources that are available to him in the community should he need help at home when the therapist is not immediately available. These resources may be suicide prevention centers, emergency rooms, ministers, and social workers. In addition, the nurse can act as a resource person in the transition from hospital to home and can talk with the patient when he returns to the hospital for outpatient care.

## CASE HISTORIES

The following are four case histories which show different types of suicidal intent, personality differences, and home situations. The nursing care is not discussed in detail in these since the subject was covered earlier in this chapter.

The first case illustrates repeated suicidal threats and gestures. The second case illustrates repeated suicidal attempts. The third case illustrates a suicidal attempt with repeated suicidal threats. The fourth case illustrates one suicidal gesture.

## Case One

Jane was 14 years old when she was admitted to the adolescent psychiatric unit. She had spent six weeks in a military hospital psychiatric unit before being transferred to our hospital. She had made three suicidal attempts with pills just prior to her hospitalization in the military hospital. She became depressed and suicidal when told she was going home; longer term hospitalization was needed, and Jane was sent to our hospital.

On admission Jane was very resistant to treatment. She would not talk with her therapist or with the staff. It took her several months to trust us (staff) and to be able to relate what her feelings were. She related better with her second therapist who was female, and was upset when she was transferred to another service. Jane was resistant with the third therapist but has since developed a very good relationship with him. She has been able to discuss with him her feelings of low self-image and worthlessness, and her problems at home of not being able to talk with her parents, and her feeling that they do not love her.

Jane has made numerous suicidal threats, gestures, and a few attempts while in the hospital. We have attempted to watch her closely and to determine her mood frequently through the day. We have moved from forcing her to have her superficial cuts cleaned and bandaged to telling her that we would like to clean them but that it is up to her when this can be done. Before the latter approach we had to struggle physically with her and thus we all (patient and staff) became upset whenever her arms had to be cleaned and bandaged.

We have tried to give Jane increased attention. Her self-mutilating behavior has greatly decreased, but she still has to be watched closely after she has contact with her family either in person, by phone, or in letters. We have spent time with Jane in activities on and off the hospital unit, using this time to get to know her and to let her get to know us.

We did not try to force her to talk about her problems but did continually let her know that we were available if she wanted to talk. She is now able to express at times what she is feeling and how she thinks we can help her. We have tried throughout Jane's stay in the hospital to let her know that we care about her, we like her, and we want to help her in any way that we can. It is very hard for her to accept the idea that people can care for her and that she is a worthy human being.

Jane's family have not been very involved in family therapy or in visiting her. We have tried on two different occasions to involve them in intense family therapy but their interest and involvement have been minimal. Jane is the last of nine children. Her father is a career man in the military but has difficulty making decisions. Her mother sets most of the limits in the home and has difficulty showing love and concern for her children. The other siblings talked with us about how they helped each other when they were growing up but Jane had no one to help her. There is little communication within the family. We feel that it would be in Jane's best interest to be placed outside the home in a group home but we are finding this difficult to accomplish since her family does not agree that she requires this. Jane herself is very ambivalent about not going home but we are trying to work through these feelings with her.

## Case Two

Diane was 16 years old when she was admitted to the adolescent psychiatric unit after making her fourth suicidal attempt. She had been hospitalized at Children's Hospital for a few hours prior to her admission for taking an overdose of 30 nembutal pills.

It was very difficult for the staff to get to know Diane. She was fighting for her independence and did not like the idea of being dependent on the hospital. However, she was able to relate with her therapist and made a lot of gains through individual therapy.

Diane lived with her mother, older sister, twin brother, and two younger sisters. Her parents were divorced two years prior to her hospitalization. When two-years-old she was allegedly involved in some incestuous relations with her father. Her mother was apparently aware of this but no action was taken. The year of the divorce Diane reported to her mother that her father had made advances toward her in a laundromat. The mother filed charges against the father but these were dropped after he went into the state hospital for a brief period of time. Shortly thereafter the mother contemplated divorce. Diane felt responsible for the divorce because of her involvement with her father.

The mother had a stroke just a few days prior to finalization of the divorce. She is partially handicapped from the stroke. Diane felt added guilt about her mother's stroke, believing herself responsible due to the added emotional stresses she had caused in the household.

Diane's mother was involved for a while in weekly therapy sessions with the social worker, but then made excuses why she could not attend and finally stopped coming. We had to contact her whenever anything came up concerning Diane's care in which it was necessary that she be involved.

During Diane's hospitalization her twin brother tried to commit suicide by pouring gasoline over himself and lighting a match. He was hospitalized at Children's Hospital on the burn unit, and was seen by a child psychiatrist from our staff. The nursing staff took Diane to Children's Hospital to visit her brother. She seemed to appreciate this since her family would not take her to see him.

Diane became a very powerful leader of the patients on the unit and it was difficult for the nursing staff to deal with her. It was felt that she had gained maximum benefit from the hospital but she could not be sent back home. She was enrolled in a program with the Bureau of Vocational Rehabilitation and in adult education classes. After leaving the hospital she completed high school. In addition, she completed a course to become a dental assistant.

After Diane left the hospital she went to live with a foster family. She had been a baby sitter for them in the past and they had expressed an interest in helping her. She had some difficult times there at first but she stayed and was able to work out her problems with them.

Diane is now working and lives in an apartment. She comes to visit us about once a year. She has mentioned often how the hospital helped her to make future plans and complete her high school education.

### Case Three

Larry is a 15 year old who was admitted to the adolescent inpatient psychiatric unit after a suicidal attempt with 100 Valium and Percodan tablets. He was hospitalized in Children's Hospital for a week and then, after psychiatric consultation, was transferred.

Larry's mother died in a car accident when he was 34 months old. He and his father were not hurt. His father became very depressed after this, and Larry was permitted to stay with relatives for a month. The father then quit his job and stayed home with Larry for a few months. After receiving encouragement from friends, Larry's father took a job and hired a housekeeper. Larry and the housekeeper liked each other and got along well. The housekeeper wanted the father to marry her and Larry knew this and probably wanted it too. The housekeeper left after six years when the father announced his plans to marry another woman. Larry was 9 years old. During the summer before his father got married, Larry's collie dog died. This was a big loss to Larry and he was never allowed to get another dog.

After Larry's father was married, he decided that all of the old household furnishings which had become rundown must be immediately removed and a new group of furnishings purchased. In retrospect, the parents wonder if this was not traumatic to Larry. In addition to the other changes, Larry's stepmother brought into the home her daughter by a previous marriage who is almost the same age as Larry.

Larry stated on admission that he had been having suicidal thoughts over the past six years since his father married. Larry and his stepmother have had many conflicts over homework, peer relationships, and so forth. He had little difficulty with his father because the father had little time to spend with him. Larry excused his father by saying he understood that he had to earn a living.

Larry was initially a very angry, withdrawn young man who denied any angry feelings. He was confronted by the staff about his negative behavior on the unit, such as his picking on other children or fighting with them. When disciplined by removal of privileges or by being sent to his room he would threaten to kill himself. Larry sometimes continued this behavior until he was put in "special care." His therapist felt that Larry engineered his going to "special care" to punish himself.

On one occasion Larry ran away from the hospital. He was followed by the male attendants. At a construction site close to the hospital, he climbed up into a building and threatened to jump. His therapist was called and upon arrival was able to talk Larry into coming down.

Larry was a difficult patient to deal with on the unit. He acted out his anger against the other patients and had to be confronted continually about his behavior. He was gradually able to decrease his hostile behavior when he began to talk in therapy about his feelings that no one cared for him and about his fears. He became supportive of staff at times before his discharge and verbalized how they had helped by setting limits on his behavior and helping him to control his anger.

Larry's suicidal leanings decreased as he was able to talk about his feelings and to relate more with his parents in family therapy. The family therapy was continued after discharge and Larry has made a good adjustment at home.

### Case Four

Susie was 15 years old when admitted to the adolescent psychiatric unit. She was transferred from Children's Hospital after a week there. She was hospitalized there after taking an unknown quantity of aspirin and penicillin, "to make me sick." She stated that she took the pills to draw attention to her home situation.

Susie has a brother who is a year older, a sister five years younger, and a brother six years younger. Her parents have been divorced for five years.

Susie's parents had been married for twelve years, but actually lived together only intermittently and probably spent a total of four years together. There were many areas of conflict in the marriage and Susie's mother was never satisfied. She left for months at a time usually taking the children with her, but then would leave them with her mother.

Mr. Jenkins, Susie's father, had to assume most of the responsibility of caring for the children. A year before the divorce, Susie's mother left the home for about a month and returned to take the children with her to Kentucky. She placed them for adoption and Mr. Jenkins was notified by the courts. He refused to place the children up for adoption and drove to Kentucky, got the children, and brought them home.

Since the divorce Mr. Jenkins had hired housekeepers and baby sitters to care for the children. Two years before her admission to the hospital, Susie asked her father not to hire any more baby sitters as she felt they were mean to the children and that she could do a better job herself. The children did have some unfortunate circumstances with the sitters in that one neglected them, another ran up large long-distance phone bills, and a third stole money from the children's banks and the household money fund.

Susie was concerned on admission because she felt that her father had been unreliable in helping to care for the younger children during the past two years. She talked on admission about her home situation and related well with others. However, she gradually withdrew and refused to talk about her home situation, refusing even to see her father or consider going home. She continued this behavior for two months. Finally Susie was able to talk about her emotional withdrawal and her past family life. She found it difficult to talk with her father in family interviews and to deal with his sporadic attendance at these. She did talk later about her father being a chronic abuser of alcohol and an unreliable parent for the children.

On the unit Susie had to learn to trust the staff. She was able, after several months, to discuss her feelings with the staff when she became depressed instead of just withdrawing into her room alone. She needed support and encouragement to participate in activities on and off the nursing unit. She did not act our her feelings against the other children, staff, or herself (by attempting to hurt herself). She needed much support to attend family interviews, and support after these when her father did not show up. She needed help and support when it was decided that legal custody should be taken from her father. Her custody was given to the Child Welfare Board. Susie was then placed with a foster family which had expressed a desire for her to live with them. They had been neighbors of the Jenkins' at one time and had kept in touch with her. Susie did well in their home after much initial support and reassurance.

## REFERENCES

1. Jacobziner H: Attempted suicides in adolescents. JAMA 191:1, Jan 4, 1965, pp 101–5
2. Bakwin H: Suicide in children and adolescents. J Pediatr 50:749–69, 1957
3. Toolan J: Suicide and suicidal attempts in children and adolescents. Am J Psychiatry 118:719–24, 1962
4. Shneidman E, Farberow N: Clues to Suicide. New York, McGraw-Hill, 1957, p 141
5. Sabbath J: The suicidal adolescent—the expendable child. Journal of the American Academy of Child Psychiatrists 8:2, 272–89, 1969
6. Schochet B: Recognizing the suicidal patient. Modern Medicine, May 18, 1970, pp 114–23
7. Editorial: Broken homes and suicide. JAMA 191:6, Feb 8, 1965, p 150
8. Peck ML: Research and training in prevention of suicide in adolescents and youth. Bulletin of Suicidology, USPHS Publ No. 6, Spring 1970, p 40
9. Seiden RH: Suicide among youth. A Supplement to the Bulletin of Suicidology, USPHS Publication, Dec 1969, p 41
10. Meeks J: The Fragile Alliance. Baltimore, Williams & Wilkins, 1971, p 205
11. Resnick HLP: Suicidal Behavior. Boston, Little, Brown, 1968, pp 299 and 300
12. Watkins C, Gilbert J, Bass W: The persistent suicidal patient. Am J Psychiatry 125:11, May 1969, p 1593
13. Brown M, Fowler G: Psychodynamic Nursing. Philadelphia, Saunders, 1966, p 203
14. Trieschman A, Whittaker J, Brendtro L: The Other 23 Hours. Chicago, Aldine, 1969, p 58
15. Schneidman E: Suicide prevention: the hospital role. Hospital Practice, Sept 1968, p 61

## BIBLIOGRAPHY

Bakwin H: Suicide in children and adolescents. J Pediatr, 50:749–69, 1957

Basler BH, Masterson JF: Suicide in adolescents. Am J Psychiatry 116:400–4, Nov 1959

Brown MM, Fowler GR: Psychodynamic Nursing. Philadelphia, Saunders, 1966

Editorial: Broken homes and suicide. JAMA 191:6, Feb 8, 1965

Jacobziner H: Attempted suicides in adolescents. JAMA 191:1, Jan 4, 1965, pp 101–05

Meeks JE: The Fragile Alliance. Baltimore, Williams & Wilkins, 1971

Peck ML: Research and training in prevention of suicide in adolescents and youth. Bulletin of Suicidology, USPHS Publ No. 6, Spring 1970, pp 35–40

Resnick HLP: Suicidal Behaviors. Boston, Little, Brown, 1968

Sabbath JC: The suicidal adolescent—the expendable child. J Am Acad Child Psychiatr 8:2, 272–89, 1969

Seiden RH: Suicide among youth. A Supplement to the Bulletin of Suicidology, USPHS Publ Dec 1969, pp 1–62

Shneidman ES: Suicide prevention: the hospital's role. Hospital Practice, Sept 1968, pp 56–61

——, Farberow NL: Clues to Suicide. New York, McGraw-Hill, 1957

Shocket BR: Recognizing the suicidal patient. Modern Medicine, May 18, 1970

Toolan JM: Suicide and suicide attempts in children and adolescents. Am J Psychiatry 118:719–24, Feb 1962

Trieschman AE, Whittaker JK, Brendtro LK: The Other 23 Hours. Chicago, Aldine, 1969

Watkins C, Gilbert JE, Bass W: The persistent suicidal patient. Am J Psychiatry 125:11, 1590–93, May 1969

# 10

# The Nurse and the Adolescent Face Death

PATRICIA A. BRANDT

"I'm fifteen.
   I'm young.
   I'm in love with life.
   I greet the dawn with a glow of enthusiasm.
   Each day brings new and exciting experiences
   And changing emotions.
I laugh
   At kittens playing
   At funny things people say,
   At foolish things I do.
I cry
   When reading a tender love story
   At disappointment too great for my youth to bear,
   For no reason at all.
I love
   The beauty of nature
   To walk barefoot through the grass with
   The wind blowing through my hair.
   The fact that I'm alive.

221

I hate
     Myself for saying and doing things that hurt
     My friends and love ones.
     I feel the pain of a broken relationship
     I worry about what people think of me.
     I think about the future.
     I ponder over my changing emotions.
     I hope for success and happiness in life.
I'm fifteen
     I'm young
     I'm in love with life. . ."[1]

What happens to this fifteen-year-old when the threat of illness and possible death slaps her in the face? What effect does the need for chemotherapy or radiation treatment have on this previously lively adolescent?

The effects of a terminal illness and treatment on the daily life of an adolescent are manyfold. The adolescent girl may be too tired from the day's classes to participate in extracurricular events. At a time when a certain amount of popularity is determined by one's appearance, the loss of long, sparkling blonde hair that took two full years to grow may be a catastrophe to the adolescent. The adolescent boy may lose the voracious appetite that previously could consume an entire pizza after a football game. The many bruises on his body may eliminate his desire to participate in the beach parties his friends have every summer. At a time when the adolescent spends hours trying to cover up facial blemishes, what must the amputation of an extremity mean to him?

All those dreams and adventures that adolescents look forward to are crushed by the threat of a terminal illness. The fantasies of being the best football player, or the most popular in the home room, or the prettiest girl at the dance, are painful to recall. It is as if "the teenager has been taken to the mountain-top and shown the panorama ahead, only to be told that the promised land is not for him."[2]

With his self-identity threatened by the loss of a body part, the adolescent finds it difficult to face his peers who previously were his primary source of communication and support. Many of an adolescent's friendships are influenced by such factors as who is the most popular at the time, who wears the latest style in clothes, or who attends all the school events. If the adolescent has a serious illness, the physical symptoms and frequent hospitalizations drastically curtail his ability and available time to participate in group activities. An adolescent's terminal illness emphasizes to his friends that sickness and possible death is real and that they may be vulnerable also. Therefore, as the adolescent's illness becomes more evident, he may gradually lose contact with friends. The friend may not be able to withstand this threat to his own identity, or the stress of having someone around who is so ill and whose presence decreases the fun and activity of the group. With the weakening of peer support, the adolescent's family again becomes, as in his earlier years, his primary support.

In many homes with a parent and adolescent under the same roof, a "mutual frustration society" typically exists. If the parent values neatness, the son will be sloppy. If the parent enjoys language that has grace, the daughter will speak slang. The adolescent talks about love and peace for members of mankind, yet recoils from motherly affection and argues with his father about hours and other privileges.[3] From these considerations it is clear that an adolescent faced with the loss of his peer group may suffer from feelings of frustration because of his dependence on his family. The adolescent, struggling with ambivalent feelings, may become bitter because of the loss of his own self-respect and independence. He may find overwhelming the penalty that life is placing on him.

Life becomes even more difficult for the adolescent who is aware that something is desperately wrong with him and yet no one is letting him in on the "secrets" of his illness and treatment. He hears his physician whisper to his parents outside his hospital room; he has been losing his hair; his brothers have stopped teasing him; his mother and father seem more solemn than ever. The adolescent may become resentful because of the lack of communication and trust demonstrated by his parents. Because the adolescent has difficulty communicating these ambivalent feelings, he may present confusing and occasionally hostile behavior to those who interact with him. A situation demonstrating this behavior occurred whenever a member of the health team would enter the hospital room of an adolescent with aplastic anemia who was receiving frequent blood transfusions. The adolescent would actively or passively attempt to degrade her mother whenever an opportunity was available. For instance, on one occasion her mother brought a record album of the daughter's favorite folk singers and the daughter threw it into the wastebasket. However, this same adolescent, when very physically weak, would insist she be bathed by her mother instead of the staff. The adolescent seemed to accept attention from her parents only when she was too physically weak to maintain her independence. Because of the variable moods and fluctuating behavior of the adolescent undergoing stress, the parent may have difficulty knowing how or when to respond to the youth's behavior.

According to Hamovitch in a study involving parents and terminally ill children of varying ages, the parents of terminally ill adolescents have more difficulty dealing with the stress of their child's illness than parents of younger children.[4] The parents recognized their adolescent's awareness of his condition, but were unable to deal with it.[4(p115)] Parents of adolescents are unable to provide the physical care or support that parents with terminally ill children ten years and under are able to provide. Parents and their adolescents may find it difficult to communicate under normal circumstances; the stress of a terminal illness certainly may compound the problem.

What then is the role of the health team member in assisting the terminally ill adolescent and his family? As a

health team member it is very important to identify one's
own concept of death before interacting with someone who
is terminally ill. Are nurses or health team members in
general comfortable when communicating about death,
especially the possibility of their own death or that of a close
family member? Is involvement of health team members with
terminally ill patients minimized by providing short and
multiple assignments in order to prevent the occurrence of
natural conversation? Are nurses consciously aware that by
prolonging contact over a period of days and even weeks with
a seriously ill adolescent, any possibility that he will initiate
efforts to talk about his concerns is definitely increased? Or
do nurses continue to play the game of mutual pretense with
the adolescent and/or his parents that nothing serious is
happening?

During a nursing report an aide related that she had
discovered Sharon, sixteen-years-old with leukemia, crying
several times this past week. No one knew what was upsetting
Sharon nor did anyone feel comfortable enough to find out.
After my spending a short time with Sharon every day for
several days talking with her about her interests and activities
at school, Sharon began crying during one of my visits. While
looking in the mirror she talked continuously about her fear
of losing all of her hair, as it had begun to fall out a week
ago. Together we talked about a solution to the problem.
Sharon remembered that a friend had recently purchased a
fall and that it looked really fashionable. During our
discussion about experimenting with different colors and
styles of both falls and wigs, Sharon seemed to relax and the
world didn't seem quite as dismal to her. Frequently, health
team members are too concerned about the types of
questions the adolescent has and whether she will ask if death
is imminent, rather than focusing on the daily, natural
concerns that are typical of the adolescent period.

When providing nursing care for a terminally ill adolescent it is essential that the adolescent's grief process and

coping behavior be understood. It is considerably important to provide a climate that will allow the family and the adolescent to progress through the grief process. The more of preparatory grief that is experienced before death, the more bearable the situation is at the time of death for both the adolescent and his family.[5] It is very difficult for a family to cope when the adolescent is killed suddenly in a car accident, as there is no time for preparatory grief. It is usually beneficial for the family and adolescent if all involved with the adolescent progress beyond the first stage of the grief process and that the grief occurs with as little guilt as possible.

According to Kubler-Ross, the first stage of the grief process is denial and isolation, or avoiding the reality of the situation.[5 (p 39)] Examples of this stage are the following: the adolescent refusing to come to the hospital for therapy; the parent talking matter-of-factly about his son's diagnosis; the adolescent writing a term paper on his diagnosis without any personal feelings included. An example of shock exhibited by a family occurred when their thirteen-year-old son was diagnosed as having osteogenic sarcoma with the necessity of leg amputation. The parents refused to make a decision until their older son received a leave from the Army. If the parents are unable to make this type of decision it may be helpful to give them a definite time period for decision making and to encourage the participation of the adolescent son who may lose his leg. To demand an immediate decision may introduce more anger and guilt than if a limited time period is given to consider all the implications.

The second stage of the grief process is anger.[5 (p 50)] Suspicion is also seen during this stage. Examples of this stage are as follows: hostility of parents toward the staff because of another exacerbation of their adolescent's illness; the adolescent accusing God or his parents for his suffering; the adolescent or parent feeling worthless and guilty; criticism of nursing care provided.

The third stage of grief is bargaining.[5](p 82) The adolescent may vow to join the missionary service if he is cured. He may plead for a few days without pain in order to play in the tennis tournament. Another example is the adolescent's nurse who says, "Let Johnny die soon, he is suffering so much. I'll be more conscientious about going to church."

Depression is the fourth stage of the grief process.[5](p 85) Depression may be evident when the adolescent has an exacerbation and is admitted to the hospital for another round of transfusions and chemotherapy. With repeated exacerbations, emotional and financial stress is increased causing the adolescent as well as his family to experience depression. One family demonstrated depression because they didn't feel free to go on a vacation for fear that the adolescent daughter would have an exacerbation of her illness during their trip.

Acceptance is the last stage of the grief process.[5](p113) The following are examples of acceptance: the parent who asks for suggestions on ways to explain the illness to the other children; the parent who becomes aware of the cues that his adolescent son is transmitting; the adolescent who asks questions about his medications. The stage of acceptance is difficult to attain and different individuals may be at different levels of acceptance. Acceptance necessarily involves a beginning emotional detachment of the family from the adolescent and the adolescent from his family. This is very heartbreaking especially when the adolescent comes closer to death and he and his family slowly detach from each other, making it somewhat less difficult for the final separation to occur.

Grief occurs as a dynamic process in which the persons involved may slip from one stage to the next at any given time, or may revert to the previous stage. For instance, a family may be reaching the stage of acceptance when the adolescent is suddenly found to have metastasis. The family at this time may demonstrate characteristics of both bargaining and anger, and yet at the same time show acceptance behaviors. It is helpful for the adolescent and his family to progress through the grief process as simultaneously as possible in order to achieve acceptance of the final reality together. Because of lack of communication, the adolescent may be in the acceptance stage while his parents remain in denial. If this occurs the adolescent may die without ever having communicated his concerns about death to his family because he was shielding them. It may be more ideal for family members to communicate with each other during stressful situations. However, individual families have previously established patterns of coping with stress and it may not be possible for them to communicate.

No matter what the family's style of coping is, the adolescent as well as his family do display intermittent periods of hope as part of the grief process. This hope may be seen, for example, when the family discusses the research being accomplished in the field of cancer. Another example of hope is the adolescent, upon his third series of chemotherapy, commenting that this time he didn't lose any more hair. An example of a parent's hope occurred when their daughter needed to have repeated thoracenteses in order to breathe, and after each of the multiple thoracenteses were performed the mother would repeatedly say, "Oh, Sherry looks so much better and her appetite has improved." Hope appears to help in meeting the demands of everyday life.

When determining the role of the individual health team members in assisting the adolescent and his family, it is important to consider how many nurses ever progress beyond the denial and isolation stage. If there is sincere interaction with the patient, the nurse may be able to progress through the grief process and be of assistance to the terminally ill adolescent and his family. It is important for the nursing staff to make the adolescent's family and friends feel welcome and significant, especially because the adolescent's attitude often creates tense and uncomfortable situations for them.

Hamovitch reports a method which enables the adolescent and his family to cope more satisfactorily with the stress of a terminal illness. When the family's home is located a distance from the inpatient facility and the adolescent is seriously ill, the family should be provided with living accommodations and meals separate from the adolescent's room.[4(p119)] Parents would be available for support and yet the adolescent's opportunity for privacy and independence would be maintained. Hamovitch also discovered that fathers had more difficulty coping after their child's death.[4(p118)] This may be related to the decreased time that fathers are able to be present during the hospitalizations and treatments for their children, which then minimizes the amount of preparatory grief experienced.

All members of the family usually benefit by participating in preparatory grief. The involvement of siblings may be to accompany the older brother to the outpatient department for his series of chemotherapy, or to visit whenever the older brother is hospitalized. Exclusion of younger siblings may increase their fantasy or guilt about the illness. It may also increase jealousy and sibling rivalry because of the noticeable increased parental attention toward the terminally ill brother or sister. The parent who constantly remains with the terminally ill adolescent may need assistance in identifying the needs of the rest of the family. For example, a mother of two younger school-age children verbally expressed her concern for the children whom she hadn't seen for two weeks. She left the bedside of her seriously ill adolescent son every two days; however, when she did go home, the other children were in school. After several alternatives were discussed with this mother, she decided to ask her son's best friend to come to visit after school every other day instead of his usual visiting time so she could be home after school. After this was arranged the school-age children would return to the hospital with the mother and father in the evenings and the father would take them home after a brief visit. This gave the entire family the opportunity to experience the grief process.

Because of the lengthy hospitalizations and multiple treatments, one of the family's concerns may be the financial burden of the adolescent's terminal illness. In order to diminish the additional stress that financial limitations place on the family, the nurse needs to be aware of and listen for these concerns, and be able to refer the family to available community resources.

Another parental concern frequently encountered was demonstrated when John's father said, "John should know he will die soon, but I just don't know what to say to him." It had been a year since John's diagnosis and the initiation of treatment; however, his parents had communicated very little to him about the illness. In this situation it was beneficial to demonstrate a method to enhance communication. Encouraging John's father to talk to him about how tired John must be, how the lumbar puncture was today, how John must miss fishing this time of year, provided a method for John's father to show his concern. About a week before John died he said to his father, "I really will die soon." John's father had never discussed death with his son but the previous days of openness enabled the father to say, "I will be with you when you need me."

In another family situation, the fourteen-year-old daughter was in the terminal phase of Hodgkin's disease. There had been no discussion of illness in this family either. Peg was a very reserved, passive adolescent who was in constant pain and yet very seldom would overtly complain. Peg's mother expressed disappointment in her own behavior toward her daughter because whenever Peg would cry out in pain, the mother would have to leave the room. Peg's mother stated, "I really want to stay but I just don't know what to do when Peg cries." With the mother present at a time when Peg was painfully uncomfortable, the nurse demonstrated to her a few measures of comfort such as holding Peg's hand, placing a cold washcloth on her forehead, and repositioning her. In a few days after continuously involving Peg's mother in this type of comforting, the mother was able to remain and support her daughter whenever she would cry out in pain.

In order to provide a climate for the family and the adolescent to progress effectively through the grief process, the following should be considered: (1) Is there consistency in staffing? (2) Are multidisciplinary team conferences planned to help the staff coordinate and cope with caring for the terminally ill? (3) Is time spent really listening for cues from the adolescent and his family? (4) Are family and friends of the adolescent encouraged to visit without constant interruptions? From the very beginning, when the adolescent is hospitalized for diagnosis, open communication must prevail. As the health team member involved with his care, a discussion of the youth's favorite songs, or sports figures may allow him to feel free to discuss other things, such as how a certain diagnostic test is performed. If the nurse encourages open communication by being open herself, the adolescent may ask her questions like: Why do the medications make me so sick if they are supposed to help? Why do I need blood again today? What is the lumbar puncture for this time? Will my hair ever grow back? How does radiation cure my problem—I've read that radiation causes cancer? During the treatment phase, the adolescent seldom asks for the hardest fact, "Am I dying?" If his questions are ignored at the beginning of his illness, too frequently the adolescent travels the road to loneliness and isolation. Since a health team member is not able to be all things to all people, the nurse should actively include in the adolescent's care the boyfriend, minister, parent, girlfriend, or whoever constitutes the adolescent's source of communication and support.

The nurse, as a health team member, is in an optimal position to observe for cues that the adolescent is ready to move out of the denial stage of the grief process. The nurse then can relate these cues to the youth's parents as well as to individual health team members involved in the care. The adolescent, parents, and health team members can then decide together the next course of action. During the adolescent's illness, the exacerbations, and remissions, it is essential that the adolescent is involved in decisions concerning his health and medical treatment.

By reliving experiences of nursing interactions with dying adolescents and their families, the grief is renewed. The stages of denial, bargaining, anger, and depression are reawakened. However, nurses are truly in an optimal position to assist these patients by providing an environment that will facilitate the progression of the family with the adolescent through the grief process. One nurse alone can not singly provide this environment. It takes several health team members cooperating with each other, and reinforcing each other when it seems too difficult to listen to one more parent's concerns.

It is worthwhile to commit oneself to involvement with dying adolescents because it may be through an individual nurse's continual effort that other health team members begin to understand how to ease the loneliness of death. And, it is especially worthwhile, when the nurse understands the full implication of the following monologue written by a dying adolescent:

> "For me, fear is today and dying is now. Don't run . . . wait . . . All I want to know is that there will be someone to hold my hand when I need it. I am afraid. Death may get to be routine to you but is new to me. Why are you afraid? I am the one who is dying."[6]

REFERENCES

1. Dicke S: Fifteen. United Church Herald 11:11, Nov 1968, p 17
2. Easson W: The Dying Child. Springfield, Ill, Charles C Thomas, 1970, p 58
3. Ginott HG: Between Parent and Teenager. New York, Macmillan, 1969, p 23
4. Hamovitch M: The Parent and the Fatally Ill Child. Duarte, Calif, City of Hope Medical Center, 1964, pp 38, 118, 119
5. Kubler-Ross E: On Death and Dying. New York, Macmillan, 1969, pp 39, 50, 82, 85, 113, 169
6. Death in the first person. Am J Nurs 70:2, Feb 1970, p 336


BIBLIOGRAPHY

Death in the first person. Am J Nurs 70:2, Feb 1970, p 336
Dicke S: Fifteen. United Church Herald 11:11, Nov 1968
Easson WM: The Dying Child. Springfield, Ill, Charles C Thomas, 1970
Ginott HG: Between Parent and Teenager. New York, Macmillan, 1969
Grollman E (ed): Explaining Death to Children. Boston, Beacon, 1967
Hamovitch M: The Parent and the Fatally Ill Child. Duarte, Calif, City of Hope Medical Center, 1964
Kubler-Ross E: On Death and Dying. New York, Macmillan, 1969
Lowenberg J: The coping behavior of fatally ill adolescents and their parents. Nurs Forum 9:3, 1970, pp 269–87

# Index